A QUICK START GUIDE TO EPI DIET COOKBOOK FOR BEGINNERS

Delicious Recipes to Eliminate Exocrine Pancreatic Insufficiency, Reduce Malabsorption, and Improve Digestion

Sarah Hayes, RD

Copyright Page

© 2024 Sarah Hayes, RD.

The recipes and information presented in this cookbook are intended for general informational purposes only. While the author and publisher have made every effort to ensure that the content is accurate and up-to-date, no guarantee is given regarding the completeness, reliability, or suitability of the information provided.

Contents

CHAPTER ONE: EXOCRINE PANCREATIC INSUFFICIENCY

Exocrine pancreatic insufficiency (EPI) is the inability to properly digest food due to a lack or reduction of digestive enzymes made by the pancreas. EPI can occur in humans and is prevalent in many conditions such as cystic fibrosis, Shwachman–Diamond syndrome, different types of pancreatitis, multiple types of diabetes mellitus (Type 1 and Type 2 diabetes), advanced renal disease, older adults, celiac disease, IBS-D, IBD, HIV, alcohol-related liver disease, Sjogren syndrome, tobacco use, and use of somatostatin analogues. EPI is caused by a progressive loss of the pancreatic cells that make digestive enzymes. Loss of digestive enzymes leads to maldigestion and malabsorption of nutrients from normal digestive processes. EPI can cause symptoms even before reaching the stages of malnutrition.

The exocrine pancreas is a portion of this organ that contains clusters of ducts (acini) producing bicarbonate anion, a mild alkali, as well as an array of digestive enzymes that together empty by way of the interlobular and main pancreatic ducts into the duodenum (upper small intestine).

The digestive enzymes serve to catalyze the breakdown of complex foodstuffs into smaller molecules for absorption and integration into metabolic pathways. The enzymes include proteases (trypsinogen and chymotrypsinogen), hydrolytic enzymes that cleave lipids, and amylase to digest starches. EPI results from progressive failure in the exocrine function of the pancreas to provide its digestive enzymes, often in response to a genetic condition or other disease state, resulting in the inability of the patient involved to properly digest food.

Causes and symptoms

What Causes EPI?

Chronic pancreatitis is the main cause of EPI in adults. As many as 8 in 10 adults with this disorder develop EPI. Pancreatitis causes inflammation and swelling of the pancreas. Over time, chronic inflammation can damage the pancreatic cells that make digestive enzymes. Doctors call this chronic pancreatitis. It happens when the enzymes made by the pancreas start working while they're still inside it, before they get to the small intestine. You're at risk for this if you're a heavy drinker, though there can be other causes as well. For instance, your pancreas could get inflamed if some passageways in it are blocked or if you have very high levels of triglycerides (a type of blood fat) or an immune system disorder. There are many reasons this can happen but some of the most common are:

You've had surgery on your pancreas, stomach, or intestines.

You have one of these inherited diseases:

Cystic fibrosis

Shwachman-Diamond syndrome

If you have cystic fibrosis, your body makes unusually thick and sticky mucus. This mucus blocks passageways in your pancreas and stops enzymes from getting out.

If you have Shwachman-Diamond syndrome, you may be missing cells in your pancreas that make enzymes.

Crohn's disease and celiac disease can also lead to EPI in some people.

Symptoms

In EPI, undigested and unabsorbed food in the digestive tract can lead to frequent gastrointestinal symptoms. Symptoms of EPI can be mild to severe and typically become more severe when 90% of your pancreas's normal enzyme production is gone. At this point, you're more likely to have symptoms clearly associated with EPI.

The hallmark symptoms of severe EPI are weight loss and loose, fatty stools called steatorrhea. While symptoms of EPI are nonspecific and can be similar to other digestive problems, it is important to ask your healthcare provider for a thorough medical evaluation if you suspect EPI. Common symptoms of EPI include:

Bloating and excessive flatulence: Bloating refers to the distension (protrusion) of the abdomen. Bloating occurs when there is too much gas or extra liquid, causing an uncomfortable feeling of tightness around the abdomen. Flatulence (passing gas) is caused by bacterial fermentation of unabsorbed foods, which releases gases like hydrogen dioxide and methane.

Abdominal pain: This can be caused by bloating and a buildup of different gases in the abdomen.

Bowel changes: This includes diarrhea and particularly foul-smelling, greasy, oily stool that is difficult to flush (steatorrhea).

Weight loss: If you have EPI, weight loss can occur even when you're eating a normal amount of food. This happens because your body is unable to break down food into smaller pieces to be absorbed as nutrients. If your body is unable to absorb nutrients like fats, you won't be able to gain weight. Malabsorption may also make your stomach feel fuller than usual, causing you to eat less and lose weight unexpectedly.

Nutritional deficiencies: Deficiencies in fat-soluble vitamins are commonly seen in people with severe forms of EPI. The inability to absorb nutrients such as fats and proteins are significant nutritional problems tied to severe EPI. You may also lack fat-soluble vitamins A, D, E, and K because they cannot be absorbed by the digestive tract. Instead, these vitamins end up being expelled from the body, along with undigested fats.

EPI and Nutritional Deficiencies

Nutritional deficiencies commonly seen in people with EPI include:

Vitamin A, which can lead to skin rashes and night blindness

Vitamin D, which can lead to low bone density such as osteopenia and osteoporosis

Vitamin E, which can increase the risk of developing macular degeneration and cataracts (clouding of the clear lens of the eye), neurological problems (depression or short-term memory loss), or muscular or joint-related issues (pain, weakness, or fatigue)

Vitamin K, which can cause abnormal bleeding or bruising.

Complications

If EPI is left untreated and becomes more severe, several complications can arise. Because complications are typically long term, they can have a significant effect on your quality of life. EPI complications may lead to skeletal, renal (kidney-related), and cardiovascular issues. These include:

Osteopenia or osteoporosis: Osteopenia is a condition in which a person's bones are weaker than what they used to be. By contrast, osteoporosis is a more severe form of osteopenia, when a person's bones are likely to break. People with severe or prolonged EPI have a vitamin D deficiency that can lead to osteopenia and may progress to osteoporosis. This is because vitamin D aids in the absorption of calcium, which is important for maintaining good bone health.

Anemia: This is a condition in which a person's red blood cells are low or are not functioning properly, causing a decrease in oxygen levels in the blood. This is caused by the malabsorption of iron or vitamin B12, which is important for making red blood cells, in people with EPI. Anemia can make a person feel weak and tired.

Heart arrhythmia: In severe cases of EPI, blood and fluid loss can leave the heart unable to pump enough blood to the body. This can lead to heart arrhythmias, which are irregular heartbeats.

Diagnosis and impact on digestion

How Is EPI Diagnosed?

Your doctor may diagnose your condition by checking your symptoms. They may ask you questions such as:

Do you have pain in your upper belly?

Have you had bad-smelling bowel movements that are oily and hard to flush down the toilet?

Do you have gas or diarrhea?

Have you lost weight?

Several tests can help diagnose EPI. First, you may need some blood tests that check to see if you're getting enough vitamins and that your pancreas is making enough enzymes. Other blood tests can check for things that can lead to EPI, like celiac disease.

You may also need to take the "3-day fecal test." It checks for the amount of fat in your bowel movements. You'll need to collect samples of your stool in special containers for 3 days.

Your doctor may also ask you to take a test called "fecal elastase-1." For this, you also need to collect a sample of your bowel movement in a container. It will be sent to a lab to look for an enzyme that's important in digestion. The test can tell you if your pancreas is making enough of it.

You may also need to get some tests that check to see if your pancreas is inflamed, including:

CT scan: This uses a powerful X-ray to make detailed pictures inside your body.

MRI: It uses strong magnets and radio waves to make pictures of organs and structures inside your body.

Endoscopic ultrasound: This test uses sound waves to take pictures inside your digestive system. The sound waves are sent out by a thin tube that your doctor places through your mouth into your digestive system.

Secretin pancreatic function test: To test how the pancreas responds to secretin, a hormone that triggers the release of digestive enzymes. For the test, you receive secretin through an intravenous (IV) line. Your provider uses endoscopic ultrasound to collect fluid and test it for enzymes.

Impact on Digestion

People with EPI can't absorb enough fats, proteins and carbohydrates from foods. This problem is called malabsorption. Your body needs these nutrients for energy and to maintain organ function. Malabsorption of nutrients can lead to malnutrition.

Signs of malnutrition include:

Dry skin, brittle nails and hair loss.

Depression.

Edema (tissue swelling).

Fatigue or dizziness.

Feeling cold all the time.

Irritability.

Memory and concentration issues.

Muscle loss.

Treatment Strategies

How Is EPI Treated?

Apart from a healthy diet, the main treatment for EPI is pancreatic enzyme replacement therapy (PERT). You take prescription pills that replace the enzymes your pancreas isn't making.

These enzymes break down your food so you can more easily digest and absorb it. You have to take them during your meals. If you take them before you eat, the replacement enzymes may move through your stomach before your food gets there. If you take the pills after you eat, you have the opposite problem.

You may also need to take an antacid to keep your stomach from breaking down pancreatic enzymes before they can start to work.

There are six FDA-approved pancreatic enzyme products that are only available by prescription:

Creon

Pancreaze

Pertzye

Ultresa

Viokace

Zenpep

If your doctor prescribes this medication, take it at the start of meals or before you eat snacks, along with a liquid like water. Don't dissolve the pill in a liquid like milk or take it with any over-the-counter stomach acid medicine that has calcium or magnesium. These products can break down the coating and enzymes in your pills.

The amount you take depends on your body weight. You'll start with the lowest possible dosage and take more if you need it.

You may also take drugs to lower stomach acid along with your PERT. Your doctor can prescribe these, and they're also available over the counter:

Proton pump inhibitors like esomeprazole or omeprazole

H2 blockers like cimetidine, famotidine, or ranitidine

You may also need medicine to treat pain. If your doctor says it's okay, you may take over-the-counter pain medicines such as acetaminophen (Tylenol) or ibuprofen (Advil, Motrin) on occasion. If those don't bring you relief, your doctor may prescribe stronger pain drugs, such as hydrocodone and oxycodone. Keep in mind that ibuprofen may lead to internal bleeding in the digestive tract and that drugs such as hydrocodone and oxycodone should be used with caution because of addiction potential.

Emotional stress can also trigger pancreas inflammation. Tricyclic antidepressants like amitriptyline or nortriptyline may help ease pain. Gabapentin (Gralise, Neurontin), a drug that helps control seizures, can also help fight EPI pain. Pregabalin (Lyrica), which is used to treat seizures and nerve pain, also shows promise.

How to Treat Conditions That Cause EPI

You also can treat the health problem that causes your EPI, like cystic fibrosis, Shwachman-Diamond syndrome, or chronic pancreatitis.

Cystic fibrosis: Treatments include enzyme replacement therapy, antibiotics, laxatives, and enemas. You can also eat a high-calorie, high-fat diet or take supplements to get the nutrition you need.

If you have cystic fibrosis and EPI, you may also get diabetes. Keep your blood sugar levels under control, and take insulin or other medications if your doctor prescribes them.

Shwachman-Diamond syndrome: Your doctor may prescribe PERTs, a high-fat and high-calorie diet, and vitamins and supplements. Scientists are also working to see if stem cell transplants will treat this genetic disease.

Chronic pancreatitis: If you have alcoholic pancreatitis, it's important to stop drinking. You may need to enter a treatment program or work with a counselor to stop. If you smoke, stop. If there are stones blocking your ducts, the doctor can remove them. If you have a systemic illness like lupus or cystic fibrosis, treatment for the underlying condition may help the chronic pancreatitis.

Is Surgery an Option?

Surgery can open ducts that are clogged or blocked by gallstones, and decompression can widen a main pancreatic duct that's too narrow.

Another option is to remove your pancreas and give you an autologous islet cell transplant. These are cells from your own body that make insulin. The doctor will get them into your body through a vein in your liver.

This surgery can ease severe chronic pancreatitis pain or prevent or ease diabetes caused by chronic pancreatitis. But it's only used if other treatments haven't worked.

If other treatments fail, the doctor might remove a portion of your pancreas, but this is usually a last resort.

CHAPTER TWO: ROLE OF DIET IN MANAGING EPI

Diet plays a large role in the management of EPI, and you should take extra care with what and how you eat. In general, you should avoid certain foods that may trigger common symptoms of EPI, which include bloating, abdominal pain, flatulence, and diarrhea. To do this, consider working with a dietitian so you can know exactly how to get proper nutrition in your meals and snacks without making your symptoms worse.

It is recommended you eat smaller meals throughout the day (to avoid bloating), avoiding too much fiber (to prevent fats from being digested), avoiding processed foods with unhealthy hydrogenated fats, and eating more lean fats (to provide your body with the fuel it needs while keeping your meals low in fat).

Key dietary considerations

1. When considering fats in your diet, it's important to choose wisely. The amount of fat recommended varies depending on factors like height, weight, and symptoms. Emphasizing the significance of fat as an essential nutrient vital for cell growth, organ protection, and body temperature regulation, experts advice against fat avoidance. Opt for fats from unsaturated sources like unsaturated oils, avocados, nuts, seeds, and fatty fish. Your healthcare provider or a registered

dietitian can assist in determining the appropriate fat intake for you.

2. Incorporate vitamins into your diet, especially if you have EPI. Supplementing with vitamins, particularly fat-soluble ones, is often necessary to prevent deficiencies. Ensuring adequate consumption of foods rich in fat-soluble vitamins A, D, E, and K is essential. Increase your intake of dark green leafy vegetables for vitamins A and K and include nuts like almonds and peanuts for vitamin E. Regular screening for vitamin deficiency is crucial, and oral supplementation may be recommended by your healthcare team based on your individual needs.

3. Prioritize omega-3 fatty acids in your diet. Individuals with EPI often have insufficient levels of essential fatty acids, increasing the risk of high triglycerides and impacting heart health. Considering an omega-3 supplement may be necessary to address this deficiency.

4. Opt for smaller, more frequent meals throughout the day instead of three large meals. Eating smaller, regular meals aids in nutrient absorption and can reduce digestive discomfort.

5. Stay hydrated by drinking plenty of water and limiting alcohol intake. Dehydration can exacerbate digestive issues, so aim for eight 8-

ounce glasses of water daily. Beverages like unsweetened tea or 100 percent fruit juice can also contribute to your hydration goals.

6. Discuss enzyme replacement therapy (ERT) with your doctor. ERT, which involves taking prescribed enzymes with meals and snacks, helps in breaking down fat and alleviating gastrointestinal symptoms. Your dietitian will assist in managing your ERT, adjusting doses based on the fat content of your meals. If weight loss persists despite ERT, dose adjustments may be necessary to improve food absorption and overall health.

EPI and fats

In the past, doctors recommended that people with EPI eat a low-fat diet. This is no longer the case because your body needs fats to absorb certain vitamins.

Avoiding fat can also make weight loss associated with EPI more severe. Taking enzyme supplements allows most people with EPI to eat a diet with normal, healthy fat levels.

When choosing meals, remember not all fats are created equal. Make sure you're getting enough essential fats. Avoid saturated and trans fats, as these can make your symptoms worse. In general, you shouldn't eat more than 20 grams of saturated fat each day or more than 10 grams of saturated fat at one meal. To do this, find ways to cut it out of your diet, like eating grilled or baked foods instead of fried foods. Also, consider using cooking spray instead of oil or butter and choosing low-fat or fat-free dairy.

Instead look for foods that contain:

monounsaturated fat

polyunsaturated fat

omega-3 fatty acids

Olive oil, peanut oil, nuts, seeds, and fish, such as salmon and tuna, all contain healthy fats.

Foods to include and avoid

Foods to eat

Most people with EPI need to eat a varied, balanced diet full of carbohydrates, fats, and protein to maintain well-being. A person can prioritize minimally processed, fresh foods whenever possible.

Lean proteins

Lean proteins, such as chicken, turkey, eggs, lentils, and fish, can provide energy while also being low in trans and saturated fats.

Healthy fats

When choosing foods high in fat, it is best to look for foods high in heart-healthy unsaturated fats. A person can limit or avoid products containing lots of saturated or trans fats.

Foods rich in healthy fats include:

nuts

seeds

olive oil

avocado

fatty fish, such as salmon

Small meals

It is best for a person with EPI to eat small, frequent meals throughout the day. This aids digestion and allows the intestines to absorb as many nutrients as possible.

Dietary supplements

Dietary supplements may help increase the nutrients a person with EPI can absorb.

Taking supplements for fat-soluble vitamins, such as A, D, E, and K, can be beneficial.

Foods to avoid

A person with EPI can aim to avoid:

high fiber foods

heavy meals

alcohol

High fiber foods

For most people, adding more fiber to the diet helps digestion and promotes a feeling of fullness. However, people living with EPI may need to limit their fiber intake. Fiber can disrupt the functioning of digestive enzymes.

A 2019 review of studies found that high fiber foods can increase the amount of fat a person loses in their stool. This may increase the risk of nutritional deficiencies.

According to some guidelines, people with EPI can avoid very high fiber diets of more than 25 grams of fiber per day.

Heavy meals

Eating larger meals can make it more difficult for the pancreas to secrete enough enzymes to adequately break down food.

People with EPI can avoid eating larger meals. Instead, they can aim to eat smaller meals more frequently throughout the day.

Alcohol

It is best for a person with EPI to avoid alcohol.

Heavy and prolonged alcohol consumption is the most common cause of chronic pancreatitis, which can lead to EPI.

Alcohol also further disrupts the production of pancreatic enzymes, which can worsen EPI symptoms.

CHAPTER THREE: PANCREATIC ENZYME REPLACEMENT THERAPY (PERT) AND DIET

PERT can help treat EPI symptoms by replacing the enzymes that your pancreas no longer makes. Through PERT, you'll receive these digestive enzymes in the form of a capsule.

The capsule enables your body to break down the proteins, fats, and carbohydrates in the foods you eat. Besides relieving the symptoms of indigestion, it can also reduce the likelihood of complications like malnutrition.

How does PERT work?

PERT capsules contain three types of digestive enzymes, which your pancreas would naturally make and release:

proteases (for digesting protein)

lipases (for digesting fats)

amylases (for digesting carbohydrates)

How to take PERT?

PERT capsules come in different units of digestive enzymes. Talk with your doctor about the specific number of units per capsule you should take.

This medication differs from other medications in that you're not prescribed a set dose per day. The general guideline is to take it right before eating, but the amount you take varies depending on your weight and how much you're eating.

For example, you might take 50,000 units or 75,000 units before dinner — the equivalent of two or three capsules. But if you're having a snack, you might only need one or two capsules before eating — the equivalent of 25,000 or 50,000 units.

The amount you'll need also depends on your level of insufficiency. You'll likely start at a lower dose (maybe 20,000 units and 40,000 units for snacks and meals, respectively).

Your doctor or dietitian can monitor your symptoms and then increase the dose as necessary. Keeping a food journal and recording your symptoms can help determine whether you need a higher amount of enzymes.

Risks and benefits of PERT

The benefits of PERT include better digestion and the reduction of EPI symptoms, such as diarrhea, constipation, and abdominal pain. But the treatment doesn't always come without risks.

Just as you might experience symptoms from insufficient enzymes, taking too much of the enzymes can also cause side effects like diarrhea and stomach pain. If symptoms don't improve after starting therapy, speak with your doctor or dietitian.

An allergic reaction to this medication is rare. Seek immediate medical care if you experience symptoms of an allergic reaction, such as:

tightness in the throat

hives

difficulty breathing

If you're allergic to pork or don't eat pork for religious reasons, be mindful that pigs are used in the preparation of these enzymes. Currently, there isn't an alternative to using pigs.

Stomach acid can destroy enzymes before they reach their target, so having too much of it — such as in cases of acid reflux or GERD — can affect how well an enzyme works.

If you're not responding to treatment, your doctor may prescribe a proton pump inhibitor (PPI), which can help reduce the production of stomach acid and are used to treat conditions such as acid reflux and GERD.

Role of enzyme supplements in EPI management

Enzyme supplements play a crucial role in managing Exocrine Pancreatic Insufficiency (EPI). Here's how they make a difference:

1. **Compensating for Insufficient Pancreatic Enzymes**: In EPI, the pancreas fails to produce adequate digestive enzymes, resulting in compromised digestion and nutrient absorption. Enzyme supplements, containing lipase, protease, and amylase, step in to aid in breaking down fats, proteins, and carbohydrates.

2. **Improving Nutrient Absorption**: Enzyme supplements bolster the breakdown of macronutrients, facilitating the absorption of vital nutrients like vitamins, minerals, and fatty acids. This is crucial for overall health, as poor absorption can lead to deficiencies and associated health issues.

3. **Alleviating Digestive Symptoms**: EPI often manifests in distressing symptoms such as bloating, abdominal pain, diarrhea, and weight loss due to undigested food traversing the digestive tract. Enzyme supplements alleviate these discomforts by enhancing digestion, reducing gastrointestinal distress, and normalizing stool consistency.

4. **Enhancing Quality of Life**: Effective EPI management with enzyme supplements

significantly improves the quality of life for those affected. By mitigating symptoms and enhancing nutritional intake, enzyme therapy empowers patients to lead fuller, more active lives unencumbered by digestive challenges.

5. **Supporting Dietary Flexibility**: Enzyme supplements grant individuals with EPI greater dietary freedom. Despite certain foods exacerbating symptoms, the use of enzyme supplements allows for a broader range of food choices without adverse effects, promoting a more varied and enjoyable diet.

6. **Tailored Dosage and Timing**: Dosage and timing of enzyme supplements are personalized based on individual needs, considering factors

such as the severity of EPI, meal size, and composition. Collaborating closely with healthcare providers ensures optimization of enzyme therapy, leading to better symptom management and nutritional well-being.

Integration of PERT with dietary habits

In addition to taking the correct unit of enzymes before meals and snacks, here are a few more tips on how to properly integrate PERT into your diet and improve how your body responds to it:

- Take capsules with a cold drink. Mixing the capsule with a hot liquid can reduce its effectiveness.

- Take the enzymes at the beginning of meals, with the first bites of food. If you wait until after the meal, the enzymes may not work properly.

- If you're taking two or three capsules with your meal, you can take one capsule at the beginning of the meal, and the other capsules at separate points through the meal.

- You should take your PERT medication if you are having a milk-based beverage. The exception is when a drink only contains a small amount of milk (such as a splash of milk in coffee or tea).

- If you have trouble swallowing the capsules, you can open the capsule and mix the granules with cold, soft acidic foods such as applesauce or gelatin. Granules should be swallowed whole and not chewed to prevent mouth sores.

- You won't need to take enzymes when eating fresh or dried fruit, or when nibbling on a small amount of vegetables.

- Don't store enzymes in hot locations, such as inside your car. This can reduce their effectiveness.

- Don't forget to take enzymes before drinking nutritional supplement drinks.

CHAPTER FOUR: DELECTABLE RECIPE IDEAS AND SUGGESTIONS YOU MUST TRY

DELECTABLE BREAKFAST IDEAS

Homemade granola

Ingredients

2 tbsp vegetable oil

125ml maple syrup

2 tbsp honey

1 tsp vanilla extract

300g rolled oats

50g sunflower seed

4 tbsp sesame seeds

50g pumpkin seeds

100g flaked almond

100g dried berries (find them in the baking aisle)

50g coconut flakes or desiccated coconut

Instructions

STEP 1

Heat oven to 150C/fan 130C/gas 2. Mix the oil, maple syrup, honey and vanilla in a large bowl. Tip in all the remaining Ingredients, except the dried fruit and coconut, and mix well.

STEP 2

Tip the granola onto two baking sheets and spread evenly. Bake for 15 mins, then mix in the coconut and dried fruit, and bake for 10-15 mins more. Remove and scrape onto a flat tray to cool. Serve with cold milk or yogurt. The granola can be stored in an airtight container for up to a month.

Eggs benedict

Ingredients

3 tbsp white wine vinegar

4 eggs

2 toasting muffins

4 parma ham

For the hollandaise sauce

125g butter

2 egg yolks

½ tsp white wine vinegar or tarragon vinegar

squeeze of lemon juice

pinch of cayenne pepper

Instructions

To prepare:

STEP 1

Bring a deep saucepan of water to the boil (at least 2 litres) and add 3 tbsp white wine vinegar. Lower the heat down to a gentle simmer.

STEP 2

Break the eggs into four separate coffee cups or ramekins. Split the muffins, toast them for a few minutes either side and warm some plates.

To make the hollandaise:

STEP 1

Melt the butter in a saucepan and skim any white solids from the surface. Keep the butter warm.

STEP 2

Put the egg yolks, white wine or tarragon vinegar, a pinch of salt and a splash of ice-cold water in a metal or glass bowl that will fit over a small pan. Whisk for a few minutes, then put the bowl over a pan of barely simmering water and whisk continuously until pale and thick, about 3-5 mins.

STEP 3

Remove from the heat and slowly whisk in the melted butter bit by bit until it's all incorporated and you have a creamy hollandaise. (If it gets too thick, add a splash of water.) Season with a squeeze of lemon juice and a little cayenne pepper. Keep warm until needed.

To make the eggs benedict:

STEP 1

Swirl the simmering vinegared water briskly to form a vortex and slide in an egg. It will curl round and set to a neat round shape. Cook for 2-3 mins, then remove with a slotted spoon.

STEP 2

Repeat with the other eggs, one at a time, re-swirling the water as you slide in the eggs. Spread some sauce on each muffin, scrunch a slice of ham on top, then top with an egg. Spoon over the remaining hollandaise and serve at once

Baked eggs brunch

Ingredients

2 tbsp olive oil

2 leeks, thinly sliced

2 onions, thinly sliced

2 x 100g bags baby spinach leaves

handful fresh wholemeal breadcrumbs

25g parmesan (or vegetarian alternative), finely grated

4 sundried tomatoes, chopped

4 medium eggs

Instructions

STEP 1

Heat oven to 200C/180C fan/gas 6. Heat the oil in a pan and add the leeks, onions and seasoning. Cook for 15-20 mins until soft and beginning to caramelise.

STEP 2

Meanwhile, put the spinach in a colander and pour over a kettle of boiling water. When cool enough to handle, squeeze out as much liquid as possible. Mix the breadcrumbs and cheese together.

STEP 3

Arrange the leek and onion mixture between 4 ovenproof dishes, then scatter with the spinach and pieces of sundried tomato. Make a well in the middle of each dish and crack an egg in it. Season and sprinkle with cheese crumbs. Put the dishes on a baking tray and cook for 12-15 mins, until the whites are set and yolks are cooked to your liking.

Leftover porridge pancakes

Ingredients

150g cold leftover porridge

150g self-raising flour

2 tsp baking powder

1 ripe banana, mashed

2 large eggs

100ml milk

2 tsp vegetable or sunflower oil

fruit, yogurt and maple syrup or honey, to serve

Instructions

STEP 1

Mix the porridge, flour, baking powder, banana, eggs and milk in a bowl. Heat the oil in a frying pan. Drop 2-3 tbsp of the porridge mixture into the pan and cook over a medium heat until the underside is golden and bubbles are popping on the surface.

STEP 2

Flip over and cook for another few mins until cooked through, then keep warm in a low oven and repeat until you've used up all the batter. Serve with the fruit and yogurt and top with a drizzle of the syrup or honey.

Veggie breakfast bakes

Ingredients

4 large field mushrooms

8 tomatoes, halved

1 garlic clove, thinly sliced

2 tsp olive oil

200g bag spinach

4 eggs

Instructions

STEP 1

Heat oven to 200C/180C fan/gas 6. Put the mushrooms and tomatoes into 4 ovenproof dishes.

Divide garlic between the dishes, drizzle over the oil and some seasoning, then bake for 10 mins.

STEP 2

Meanwhile, put the spinach into a large colander, then pour over a kettle of boiling water to wilt it. Squeeze out any excess water, then add the spinach to the dishes. Make a little gap between the vegetables and crack an egg into each dish. Return to the oven and cook for a further 8-10 mins or until the egg is cooked to your liking.

Red velvet pancakes

Ingredients

200g self raising flour

2 tbsp cocoa powder

1 tsp baking powder

1 tbsp golden caster sugar

½ tsp vanilla extract

230ml milk

3 eggs

25g butter, melted plus extra for frying

red gel food colouring

For the toppings

100g cream cheese

4 tbsp maple syrup

100g chocolate chips

icing sugar, for dusting

handful blueberries (optional)

Instructions

STEP 1

Mix all of the pancake Ingredients (except the food colouring) together in a large bowl, whisk thoroughly until smooth. Now add a small amount of red food colouring and mix again. Add more colouring until the batter is a rich reddish brown.

STEP 2

Put a small knob of butter in a large non-stick frying pan over a medium-low heat and cook until melted and foaming. Pour 2 tbsp of the mixture into the pan and use the back of the spoon to shape it into a 8-9cm round disc. Depending on the size of your pan you may be able to get 2 or 3 pancakes to cook at the same time. Cook for 2-3 mins on the first side, then flip over and cook for another 1 min on the other.

STEP 3

Heat oven to its lowest setting and stack up the cooked pancakes on a baking tray to keep warm in the oven while you cook the rest. In a small bowl mix together the cream cheese and maple syrup then set aside until needed. To serve, stack the pancakes with the cream cheese mixture and chocolate chips in between them then finish with a final dollop of the cream cheese, a dusting of icing sugar and a few fresh blueberries if you like.

Almond flour pancakes

Ingredients

2 eggs

60ml almond milk

1 tbsp maple syrup

125g almond flour

1 tsp baking powder

1 tsp vanilla extract

blueberries, to serve

Instructions

STEP 1

Whisk together the eggs, almond milk and maple syrup, then tip in the almond flour, baking powder, ¼ tsp salt and the vanilla, and stir together.

STEP 2

Heat a non-stick frying pan over a medium-low heat. Add a couple of heaped tablespoons of the batter and cook until the edges are set, around 2-3 mins. Flip and cook for a further 2 mins until golden. Repeat with the remaining batter. Serve the pancakes in small stacks, scattered with the blueberries.

Ham & potato hash with baked beans & healthy 'fried' eggs

Ingredients

600g potato, diced

1 Cal cooking spray, for frying

2 leeks, trimmed, washed and sliced

175g lean ham, weighed after trimming and discarding any fat, chopped

2 tbsp wholegrain mustard

5 eggs

2 x 415g cans reduced sugar & salt baked beans

Instructions

STEP 1

Bring a large pan of salted water to the boil. Add the potatoes and boil for 5 mins until just tender. Drain well and leave in the colander to steam-dry.

STEP 2

Meanwhile, spray an ovenproof pan with cooking spray. Add the leeks with a splash of water and fry until very soft and squishy. Add a few more sprays of the oil, tip in the potatoes along with the ham, and fry to crisp up a little. Heat oven to 200C/180C fan/gas 6.

STEP 3

Stir in the mustard, 1 egg and a good amount of seasoning with a fork – break up some of the potatoes roughly as you do. Flatten down the mixture, spray the top with oil, and bake in the oven for 15-20 mins until the top is crisp.

STEP 4

When the hash is nearly ready, heat 200ml water in a non-stick frying pan with a lid (or use a baking sheet as a lid). When it is steaming (but before it simmers), crack in the remaining 4 eggs and cover with a lid. Cook for 2-4 mins until the eggs are done to your liking. Meanwhile, heat the beans.

STEP 5

Lift an egg onto each plate, add a big scoop of hash and spoon on some beans.

Breakfast burrito

Ingredients

1 tsp chipotle paste

1 egg

1 tsp rapeseed oil

50g kale

7 cherry tomatoes, halved

½ small avocado, sliced

1 wholemeal tortilla wrap, warmed

Instructions

STEP 1

Whisk the chipotle paste with the egg and some seasoning in a jug. Heat the oil in a large frying pan, add the kale and tomatoes.

STEP 2

Cook until the kale is wilted and the tomatoes have softened, then push everything to the side of the pan. Pour the beaten egg into the cleared half of the pan and scramble. Layer everything into the centre of your wrap, topping with the avocado, then wrap up and eat immediately

Creamy mushrooms on toast

Ingredients

1 slice wholemeal bread

1 ½ tbsp light cream cheese

1 tsp rapeseed oil

3handfuls sliced, small flat mushrooms

2 tbsp skimmed milk

¼ tsp wholegrain mustard

1 tbsp snipped chives

Instructions

STEP 1

Toast the bread, then spread with a little of the cream cheese.

STEP 2

Meanwhile, heat the oil in a non-stick pan and cook the mushrooms, stirring frequently, until softened. Spoon in the milk, remaining cheese and the mustard. Stir well until coated. Tip onto the toast and top with chives.

Sweet potato pancakes with orange & grapefruit

Ingredients

325g sweet potatoes, peeled and coarsely grated

½ tsp vanilla extract

2 oranges, 1 zested, both cut into segments

150g ricotta or bio yogurt

2 large eggs

½ tsp baking powder

2 tsp rapeseed oil

2 grapefruits, cut into segments

small handful mint leaves

Instructions

STEP 1

Put the sweet potato in a bowl, cover with cling film and cook in the microwave on high for 5 mins (or steam them). Mash the potato with a fork. When cooled a little, beat in the vanilla, orange zest, ricotta, eggs and baking powder to make a batter.

STEP 2

Heat the oil in a non-stick frying pan and fry spoonfuls of the batter for a few mins. Carefully flip the pancakes to cook the other side. When done, set aside on a plate and cook the remaining batter, aiming for eight pancakes in total.

Chocolate-orange French toast

Ingredients

4 thick slices of brioche, challah or panettone

2 tbsp marmalade

40g dark chocolate, broken into pieces

3 eggs

300ml whole milk

1 tsp vanilla extract

1 orange, zested, then peeled and sliced

¼ tsp ground cinnamon

2 tbsp unsalted butter

2 tbsp maple syrup

icing sugar, for dusting

yogurt or crème fraîche, to serve

Instructions

STEP 1

Heat the oven to 140C/120C fan/gas 1. Cut a pocket into the side of each thick slice of bread using a small, sharp knife, then spoon in a quarter of the marmalade and poke a quarter of the chocolate into each pocket.

STEP 2

Whisk the eggs, milk, vanilla, orange zest and cinnamon together in a shallow dish. Dip each slice of bread into the egg mixture, making sure both sides are fully coated.

STEP 3

Melt ½ tbsp of the butter in a large frying pan over a medium heat. Lay a soaked bread slice in the pan and cook until golden brown and crispy, about 2-3 mins per side. Repeat with the remaining slices.

Keep the toasted slices warm in a low oven while cooking the next, adding more butter as needed.

STEP 4

Put the orange slices in a pan with the maple syrup and warm through over a low-medium heat until some of their juices are released. Dust the French toast with icing sugar and top with the yogurt, orange slices and warm maple-orange syrup.

Blueberry baked oats

Ingredients

500ml almond milk

200g jumbo porridge oats

2 tbsp almond butter

1 tsp baking powder

1 egg, beaten

1 small ripe banana, mashed

½ tsp almond extract or 1 tsp vanilla extract (optional)

450g blueberries, plus extra to serve

30g whole, skin-on almonds, roughly chopped

milk or fat-free yogurt and honey, to serve (optional)

Instructions

STEP 1

Heat the oven to 200C/180C fan/gas 6. Mix all of the Ingredients together in a large bowl.

STEP 2

Tip the mixture into a 2-litre ovenproof dish, then
bake for 30-35 mins until piping hot in the middle.
Serve warm with a little milk or yogurt, honey and
extra blueberries, if you like.

Belgian waffles

Ingredients

240ml buttermilk

60g unsalted butter, melted

½ tsp vanilla extract

1 large egg

240g plain flour

½ tsp salt

1 tbsp caster sugar

½ tsp baking powder

¼ tsp bicarbonate of soda

oil, for greasing

Serving suggestions

berries, Greek yogurt and a drizzle of honey, streaky bacon and maple syrup, ice cream and chocolate sauce, peanut butter and banana

Instructions

STEP 1

Whisk the buttermilk, melted butter and vanilla together in a large bowl. Separate the egg and whisk the yolk into the buttermilk mixture. Whisk the egg white in a clean bowl until it forms stiff peaks – this will keep your waffles light and fluffy.

STEP 2

Sift all the dry Ingredients into a bowl. Whisk in the wet Ingredients to create a smooth batter then carefully but decisively fold through the egg white – don't worry if you are left with a few small lumps. Cover with cling film and leave the batter to sit for 30 mins, if you have time.

Cinnamon crêpes with nut butter, sliced banana & raspberries

Ingredients

75g gluten-free brown bread flour

1 tsp ground cinnamon

1 medium egg

225ml semi-skimmed milk

1 tsp rapeseed oil, for frying

2 tbsp almond nut butter (make your own with recipe in 'goes well with', right)

1 banana, sliced

140g raspberries

lemon wedges

Instructions

STEP 1

Tip the flour into a large mixing bowl with the cinnamon. Add the egg and milk, and whisk vigorously until you have a smooth pouring consistency.

STEP 2

Place a non-stick frying pan over a medium heat and add a little of the oil. When the oil starts to heat, wipe most of it away with kitchen paper. Once the pan is hot, pour a small amount of the batter into the centre of the pan and swirl it to the sides of the pan in a thin layer. Leave to cook, untouched, for about 2 mins. When it is brown underneath, turn over and cook for 1 min more.

STEP 3

Transfer to a warm plate and cover with foil to keep warm. Repeat with the remaining batter. Divide the warm pancakes between 2 plates and serve with the nut butter, banana, raspberries and lemon to assemble at the table.

DELECTABLE LUNCH IDEAS

Easy salmon sushi rice bowl

Ingredients

150g sushi rice

pinch of caster sugar

1 tbsp rice vinegar

120g frozen edamame

1 large carrot

handful of radishes

¼ cucumber

2 cooked skinless salmon fillets

1-2 tbsp soy sauce

1 tsp toasted sesame seeds

few pieces of sushi ginger, optional

Equipment

scales

measuring jug

medium saucepan with a lid

measuring spoons

wooden spoon

small saucepan

vegetable peeler

chopping board

sharp knife

Directions

STEP 1

Tip the sushi rice into a medium saucepan, cover with 200ml water and add a pinch of salt. Put the pan on the hob and turn the heat to high. Wait for the water to boil, then reduce the heat to very low, cover the pan with a lid and leave to gently cook for 15 mins.

STEP 2

After 15 mins turn off the heat, fluff up the rice with a fork, then return the lid to the pan and leave for another 5 mins, the rice will continue to cook. After 5 mins, check the rice is cooked – it should have absorbed all the water and be soft but not mushy. Stir the sugar and vinegar through the rice, cover with the lid again and leave to keep warm while you prepare the other Ingredients.

STEP 3

Fill a small pan halfway with water, put it on the hob and bring the water to a gentle boil. Add the edamame beans, cook for 3 mins, and then carefully drain.

STEP 4

Peel the carrot and discard the outer skin, then keep peeling the flesh to create lots of carrot ribbons.

STEP 5

Thinly slice the radishes. Cut the cucumber into batons, then thinly slice lengthways.

STEP 6

With your hands, break the salmon into small pieces – look out for any bones and throw these away.

STEP 7

Divide the warm rice between two bowls and arrange the other Ingredients on top, then drizzle with the soy sauce and sesame seeds, and add a few pieces of sushi ginger, if using.

Harissa chicken with chickpea salad

Ingredients

250g punnet cherry tomatoes, halved

½ small red onion, chopped

400g can chickpeas, drained

small bunch parsley, roughly chopped

juice 1 lemon

2 skinless chicken breasts, halved lengthways through the middle

1 tbsp harissa

fat-free natural yogurt and wholemeal pitta bread, to serve

Directions

STEP 1

Mix the tomatoes, onion and chickpeas together, stir through the parsley and lemon juice and season.

STEP 2

Coat the chicken with the harissa. Heat a griddle or frying pan or barbecue. Cook the chicken for 3-4 mins each side until lightly charred and cooked through.

STEP 3

Divide the salad between 2 plates, top with the harissa chicken and serve with a dollop of yogurt and warmed pitta bread.

Spicy fish stew

Ingredients

1 tbsp olive oil

2 onions, thinly sliced

3 spring onions, chopped

3 garlic cloves, chopped

1 red chilli, seeded and thinly sliced

few thyme sprigs

2 x 400g cans chopped tomatoes

400ml vegetable bouillon made with 2 tsp vegetable bouillon powder

2 green peppers, seeded and cut into pieces

160g brown basmati rice

400g can and 210g can red kidney beans, drained

handful fresh coriander, chopped, plus a few sprigs extra

handful flat-leaf parsley, chopped

550g pack frozen wild salmon, skinned and cut into large pieces

1 lime, zested

Directions

STEP 1

Heat the oil in a large non-stick pan and fry the onions for 8-10 mins until softened and golden. Add the spring onions, garlic, chilli and thyme. Cook, stirring, for 1 min. Pour in the tomatoes and bouillon, then stir in the peppers. Cover and leave to simmer for 15 mins.

STEP 2

Meanwhile, cook the rice according to pack instructions. Stir in the beans with the coriander and parsley, then leave to cook gently for another 10 mins until the peppers are tender. Add the salmon and lime zest and cook for 4-5 mins until cooked through.

STEP 3

Ladle into bowls and scatter with the coriander sprigs.

Chicken & avocado salad with blueberry balsamic dressing

Ingredients

1 garlic clove

85g blueberries

1 tbsp extra virgin rapeseed oil

2 tsp balsamic vinegar

125g fresh or frozen baby broad beans

1 large cooked beetroot, finely chopped

1 avocado, stoned, peeled and sliced

85g bag mixed baby leaf salad

175g cooked chicken

Directions

STEP 1

Finely chop the garlic. Mash half the blueberries with the oil, vinegar and some black pepper in a large salad bowl.

STEP 2

Boil the broad beans for 5 mins until just tender. Drain, leaving them unskinned.

STEP 3

Stir the garlic into the dressing, then pile in the warm beans and remaining blueberries with the beetroot, avocado, salad and chicken. Toss to mix, but don't go overboard or the juice from the beetroot will turn everything pink. Pile onto plates or into shallow bowls to serve.

Broccoli pesto & pancetta pasta

Ingredients

300g head broccoli, broken into florets

300g pasta (we used orecchiette)

1 tbsp pine nuts

1 large bunch of basil

1 large garlic clove

2 tbsp parmesan, finely grated

1 tbsp olive oil

50g smoked pancetta, diced

200g cherry tomatoes, halved

Directions

STEP 1

Bring a pan of lightly salted water to the boil. Add the broccoli and boil for 5 mins. Scoop out with a slotted spoon and set aside.

STEP 2

Put the pasta in the same pan and cook following pack instructions. Meanwhile, tip the broccoli into a food processor with the pine nuts, basil, garlic, parmesan and oil, and blitz until smooth. Season with black pepper and a little salt (the pancetta is very salty).

STEP 3

Set a frying pan over a medium heat and cook the pancetta for 2 mins. Add the tomatoes and cook for 3 mins, or until softened. Toss the pasta with the broccoli pesto, tomatoes and pancetta, and loosen with a splash of pasta water, if needed. Spoon into bowls and serve.

Mexican-style stuffed peppers

Ingredients

3 large mixed peppers, halved

oil, for drizzling

2 x 250g pouches lime & coriander rice, cooked

400g can black beans, drained and rinsed

6 Mexican-style chilli cheese slices (use regular cheddar or monterey jack, if you like)

150g fresh guacamole

Directions

STEP 1

Heat the oven to 220C/200C fan/gas 7 or preheat the air fryer to 180C for 4 mins.

STEP 2

Remove the seeds and any white pith from the peppers and arrange them, cut-side up, in a roasting tin for the oven or in the air fryer basket for the air fryer. In both cases, brush the peppers with oil and season them.

STEP 3

If using the oven, bake the peppers for 20 mins. If using the air-fryer, cook the peppers in a single layer for 8-10 mins until they are softened and starting to caramelise.

STEP 4

Combine the rice and beans.

STEP 5

For the oven method, remove the peppers from the oven and fill them with the rice mixture. Top each with a slice of cheese and bake for an additional 10-15 mins, until the cheese has melted, and the filling is hot.

STEP 6

For the air-fryer method, remove the peppers from the air-fryer and fill them with the rice mixture. Top each with a slice of cheese and air-fry for 3 mins more, until the cheese has melted and the filling is hot.

Mushroom risotto

Ingredients

50g dried porcini mushrooms

1 vegetable stock cube

2 tbsp olive oil

1 onion, finely chopped

2 garlic cloves, finely chopped

250g pack chestnut mushrooms, chopped

300g risotto rice, such as arborio

1 x 175ml glass white wine

25g butter

handful parsley leaves, chopped

50g parmesan or Grana Padano, freshly grated

Directions

STEP 1

Put 50g dried porcini mushrooms into a large bowl and pour over 1 litre boiling water. Soak for 20 mins, then drain into a bowl, discarding the last few tbsp of liquid left in the bowl.

STEP 2

Crumble 1 vegetable stock cube into the mushroom liquid, then squeeze the mushrooms gently to remove any liquid.

STEP 3

Heat 2 tbsp olive oil in a shallow saucepan or deep frying pan over a medium flame. Add 1 finely chopped onion and 2 finely chopped garlic cloves, then fry for about 5 mins until soft.

STEP 4

Stir in 250g chopped chestnut mushrooms and the dried mushrooms, season with salt and pepper and continue to cook for 8 mins until the fresh mushrooms have softened.

STEP 5

Tip 300g risotto rice into the pan and cook for 1 min. Pour over a 175ml glass of white wine and let it bubble to nothing so the alcohol evaporates.

STEP 6

Keep the pan over a medium heat and pour in a quarter of the mushroom stock. Simmer the rice, stirring often, until the rice has absorbed all the liquid.

STEP 7

Add about the same amount of stock again and continue to simmer and stir - it should start to become creamy, plump and tender. By the time the final quarter of stock is added, the rice should be almost cooked.

STEP 8

Continue stirring until the rice is cooked. If the rice is still undercooked, add a splash of water. Take the pan off the heat, add 25g butter and scatter over 25g grated parmesan or Grana Padano cheese and half a handful of chopped parsley leaves.

STEP 9

Cover and leave for a few mins so that the rice can take up any excess liquid as it cools a bit. Give the risotto a final stir, spoon into bowls and scatter with the remaining 25g grated cheese and the remaining chopped parsley leaves.

Quick and easy fish stew

Ingredients

1 tbsp olive oil

1 tsp fennel seeds

2 carrots, diced

2 celery sticks, diced

2 garlic cloves, finely chopped

2 leeks, thinly sliced

400g can chopped tomatoes

500ml hot fish stock, heated to a simmer

2 skinless pollock fillets (about 200g), thawed if frozen, and cut into chunks

85g raw shelled king prawns

Directions

STEP 1

Heat the oil in a large pan, add the fennel seeds, carrots, celery and garlic, and cook for 5 mins until starting to soften. Tip in the leeks, tomatoes and stock, season and bring to the boil, then cover and simmer for 15-20 mins until the vegetables are tender and the sauce has thickened and reduced slightly.

STEP 2

Add the fish, scatter over the prawns and cook for 2 mins more until lightly cooked. Ladle into bowls and serve with a spoon.

Vegetarian fajitas

Ingredients

400g can black beans, drained

small bunch coriander, finely chopped

4 large or 8-12 small flour tortillas

1 avocado, sliced, or 1 small tub guacamole

2 tbsp soured cream or crème fraîche

For the fajita mix

1 red and 1 yellow pepper, cut into strips

1 tbsp oil

1 red onion, cut into thin wedges

1 garlic clove, crushed

½ tsp chilli powder

½ tsp smoked paprika

½ tsp ground cumin

1 lime, juiced

Directions

STEP 1

To make the fajita mix, take two or three strips from each colour of pepper and finely chop them. Set aside. Heat the oil in a frying pan and fry the remaining pepper strips and the onion until soft and starting to brown at the edges. Cool slightly and mix in the chopped raw peppers. Add the garlic and cook for 1 min, then add the spices and stir. Cook for a couple of mins more until the spices become aromatic, then add half the lime juice and season. Transfer to a dish, leaving any juices behind, and keep warm.

Chicken tacos

Ingredients

250g plain flour, plus extra for dusting

2 tbsp rapeseed oil

2 tbsp taco or fajita seasoning (see tip, below)

5-6 skinless chicken breasts, sliced

¼ red cabbage, finely shredded

3 limes, 1 juiced, 2 cut into wedges

small bunch of coriander, chopped

4 sweetcorn cob, kernels sliced off, or 400g frozen sweetcorn

400g can black beans, drained and rinsed

2 garlic cloves, crushed

4 tbsp fat-free yogurt, to serve

chilli sauce, to serve

Directions

STEP 1

Combine the flour with half the oil and a small pinch of salt in a bowl. Pour over 125-150ml warm water, then bring together into a soft dough with your hands. Cut into six equal pieces, then cut four of the pieces in half again, so you have eight small pieces and two large. Roll all the pieces out on a floured work surface until they're as thin as you can get them.

STEP 2

Heat a dry frying pan over a medium-high heat and cook the small and large tortillas for 2-3 mins on each side until golden and toasted (do this one at a time). Leave the large tortillas to cool, then cover and reserve for use in the lunchboxes (see tip below). Keep the small tortillas warm in foil.

STEP 3

Sprinkle the taco seasoning over the chicken in a bowl, and toss to combine. Toss the cabbage with the lime juice, half the coriander and some seasoning in another bowl, then leave to pickle.

STEP 4

Meanwhile, heat two frying pans over a high heat. Divide the remaining oil between the pans and fry the sweetcorn and a pinch of salt until sizzling and turning golden, stirring occasionally – you want the sweetcorn to char slightly, as this adds flavour, so you may need to leave it to cook undisturbed for a bit. While the sweetcorn cooks and chars, fry the chicken in the larger pan until cooked through and golden (you may need to do this in batches).

STEP 5

Tip the black beans and garlic into the sweetcorn and stir to warm through. Squeeze over two of the lime wedges.

STEP 6

Reserve two spoonfuls each of the chicken (about 1 chicken breast) and sweetcorn mix for use in the lunchboxes (see tip, below), then serve the rest in bowls alongside the cabbage, yogurt, lime wedges, remaining coriander, chilli sauce and tortillas for everyone to dig into.

Easy risotto with bacon & peas

Ingredients

1 onion

2 tbsp olive oil

knob of butter

6 rashers streaky bacon, chopped

300g risotto rice

1l hot vegetable stock

100g frozen peas

freshly grated parmesan, to serve

Directions

STEP 1

Finely chop 1 onion. Heat 2 tbsp olive oil and a knob of butter in a pan, add the onions and fry until lightly browned (about 7 minutes).

STEP 2

Add 6 chopped rashers streaky bacon and fry for a further 5 minutes, until it starts to crisp.

STEP 3

Add 300g risotto rice and 1l hot vegetable stock, and bring to the boil. Stir well, then reduce the heat and cook, covered, for 15-20 minutes until the rice is almost tender.

STEP 4

Stir in 100g frozen peas, add a little salt and pepper and cook for a further 3 minutes, until the peas are cooked.

STEP 5

Serve sprinkled with freshly grated parmesan and freshly ground black pepper.

Vitality chicken salad with avocado dressing

Ingredients

handful frozen soya beans

1 skinless cooked chicken breast, shredded

¼ cucumber, peeled, deseeded and chopped

½ avocado, flesh scooped out

few drops Tabasco sauce

juice ½ lemon, plus a lemon wedge

2 tsp extra-virgin olive oil

5-6 Little Gem lettuce leaves

1 tsp mixed seed

Directions

STEP 1

Blanch the soya beans for 3 mins. Rinse in cold water and drain thoroughly. Put the chicken, beans and cucumber in a bowl.

STEP 2

Blitz the avocado, Tabasco, lemon juice and oil in a food processor or with a hand blender. Season, pour into the bowl and mix well to coat.

STEP 3

Spoon the mixture into the lettuce leaves (or serve it alongside them) and sprinkle with the seeds. Chill until lunch, then serve with a lemon wedge.

Scotch broth

Ingredients

250g broth mix (or a mixture of 75g pearl barley, 75g yellow split peas, 50g red split lentils and 50g green split or marrowfat peas)

1 tbsp vegetable or olive oil

1 large onion, finely chopped

1 leek, washed and sliced

1 medium turnip, peeled and finely chopped

3 carrots, finely chopped

3 celery sticks, trimmed and finely chopped

3 litres lamb stock

200g kale chopped

Directions

STEP 1

Rinse the soup mix and soak in cold water for 8 hrs or overnight, covered in a cool place. Drain and rinse well.

STEP 2

Heat the oil in a large pan and fry the onion, leek, turnip, carrots and celery for 10 mins, covered with a lid, until soft but not golden. Add a generous pinch of salt and a good grinding of pepper.

STEP 3

Pour the stock into the pan and bring to a simmer. Add the drained soup mix, and gently simmer for 1 hr part-covered, until the barley and split peas are tender. Season again if needed. Stir in the kale, and cook for 10-15 mins until tender, then ladle into bowls to serve.

Moroccan-style chickpea soup

Ingredients

1 tbsp olive oil

1 onion, chopped

2 celery sticks, chopped

2 tsp ground cumin

600ml hot vegetable stock

400g can chopped plum tomatoes with garlic

400g can chickpeas, rinsed and drained

100g frozen broad beans

zest and juice ½ lemon

large handful coriander or parsley and flatbread, to serve

Directions

STEP 1

Heat the oil in a large saucepan, then fry the onion and celery gently for 10 mins until softened, stirring frequently. Tip in the cumin and fry for another min.

STEP 2

Turn up the heat, then add the stock, tomatoes and chickpeas, plus a good grind of black pepper. Simmer for 8 mins. Throw in broad beans and lemon juice, cook for a further 2 mins. Season to taste, then top with a sprinkling of lemon zest and chopped herbs. Serve with flatbread

One pot chicken and mushroom risotto

Ingredients

50g butter

85g smoked bacon lardons

1 large onion, halved and finely chopped

250g chestnut mushrooms, thickly sliced

300g arborio risotto rice

150ml dry white wine

1.4l hot chicken stock

140g cooked chicken, chopped

50g grated parmesan, plus extra to serve (optional)

½ small pack of flat-leaf parsley, chopped

Directions

STEP 1

Heat the butter in a large pan. Add the lardons and fry for 5 mins over a low-medium heat. Stir in the onion and fry for 10 mins more until the onion is soft but not coloured.

STEP 2

Stir in the mushrooms and continue cooking, stirring, for 5 mins. Stir in the risotto rice and cook over a medium heat for 2 mins until the rice has started to turn translucent.

STEP 3

Pour in the wine and allow it to bubble away over the heat. Pour in a quarter of the chicken stock and set a timer for 20 mins.

STEP 4

Continue cooking, stirring very frequently, topping up with a splash more stock as it gets absorbed – this is best done in three more stages, until the rice is cooked and most of the stock has been absorbed (you may not need all the stock). The texture now should be creamy, like rice pudding.

STEP 5

Stir through the chicken, warm briefly, then turn off the heat. Stir through the parmesan and parsley, cover and leave to rest for 5 mins to allow more liquid to be absorbed into the rice. Season to taste and serve with extra parmesan, if you like.

DELECTABLE DINNER IDEAS

Chicken tikka

Ingredients

3 large chicken breasts, cut into chunks

75g Greek yogurt

2 tbsp ginger and garlic paste

1 tbsp madras curry powder

1 tsp ground cumin

1 tsp ground coriander

1 tsp ground turmeric

1 tsp smoked paprika

2 tsp mild chilli powder

1 tbsp lemon juice

Directions

STEP 1

Tip all of the Ingredients into a large bowl with a big pinch of salt and pepper and mix well. Cover and chill for at least a few hours, but preferably overnight.

STEP 2

Heat the grill or a barbecue to high. Thread the chicken pieces onto four metal skewers, packing the pieces in so they're all touching. Put onto a baking tray under the grill, or onto the grills of the barbecue and cook for 4-5 mins, until charred, then flip and repeat.

Baked chicken breast with spice mix seasoning

Ingredients

4 chicken breasts (skinless, if you like)

1½ tbsp light brown soft sugar

1½ tsp paprika

1 tsp dried thyme

1 tsp dried oregano

¼ tsp garlic granules

½ tsp sea salt

potato wedges and green veg, to serve (optional)

Directions

STEP 1

Heat the oven to 180C/160C fan/gas 4. Arrange the chicken breasts (skin-side up, if not using skinless) in a baking tray or dish lined with baking parchment. Combine the sugar, spices, herbs, salt and ½ tsp freshly ground black pepper, then spoon a quarter of the spice mix over each chicken breast and rub it all over the meat.

STEP 2

Bake the chicken breasts for 25-30 mins until cooked through – the spice mix coating will darken and the sugar will caramelise. Serve the chicken with potato wedges and green veg, if you like.

Bigos (Polish hunter's stew)

Ingredients

1 white cabbage finely sliced

250ml beef stock

100g dried mushrooms, soaked in boiling water for 1 hr

2 tbsp lard

400g German-style sausages, sliced

250g smoked bacon, diced or sliced

2 onions, chopped

750g cooked pork, game meat or beef, diced

200g prunes

1 bay leaf

2 cloves

12 peppercorns

4 juniper berries

4 allspice berries

90ml red wine

2 tbsp tomato purée

Directions

STEP 1

Put the cabbage in a heavy casserole dish, add the stock and cook over a low heat for about 50 mins, until tender.

STEP 2

Cut the soaked mushrooms into strips and save the soaking water. Heat the lard and fry the sausages and bacon, then scoop out, leaving the fat in the pan. Fry the onion in the same pan for 5-8 mins until lightly browned.

STEP 3

Add the mushrooms and their liquid along with all the cooked meat, onions and prunes, then cover and cook for 20 mins. Add the spices, red wine and tomato purée and bring to a simmer, then cover and cook for 1 hr. Season well and leave to cool. Will keep covered and chilled for up to two days. Bigos improves in flavour over a couple of days. Leave to cool first. Reheat until piping hot before serving.

Meat & potato pie

Ingredients

2 tbsp vegetable or sunflower oil

1.2kg stewing steak, cut into chunks

2 onions, sliced

2 bay leaves

2 thyme or rosemary sprigs

750ml beef stock

750g Maris Piper potatoes, halved, quartered if large

1-2 tsp cornflour

320g pack ready-rolled shortcrust pastry, or 500g
block shortcrust pastry

plain flour, for dusting

1 egg, beaten

Directions

STEP 1

Heat the oil in a large lidded pan over a medium
heat and brown the meat well all over (you may
need to do this in batches). This will take 20-25
mins. Remove to a plate and set aside.

STEP 2

Fry the onions in the pan for 3-4 mins until starting
to brown, then return the meat to the pan and add
the bay leaves and thyme or rosemary. Pour in the

stock and bring to a simmer. Cook for 1 hr 30 mins-2 hrs, checking every 30 mins until the meat is tender.

STEP 3

Tip in the potatoes and cook for 10-12 mins more until the potatoes are just cooked through. Remove 2 tbsp liquid from the pan and combine with the cornflour to make a paste, then pour this back into the mixture, stir and simmer until thickened. Remove from the heat and tip the filling into a large ovenproof dish.

STEP 4

Heat the oven to 200C/180C fan/gas 6. Roll the pastry out on a lightly floured surface into a rectangle the thickness of a 50p piece large enough to cover the dish. Lay the pastry rectangle over the dish and crimp it around the rim of the dish to seal, trimming any excess. Cut two holes in the top of the pastry to allow any steam to escape, then brush over the beaten egg. Bake for 20-30 mins until the pastry is golden. Leave to rest for a few minutes, then serve hot.

Ukrainian pork rib borsch

Ingredients

1.5kg pork ribs

2 onions

1 medium beetroot, peeled and cut into matchsticks

2 tbsp vegetable oil (optional)

2 medium carrots, grated

4 medium potatoes, chopped

2 tbsp tomato purée

400g can chopped tomatoes

1 bay leaf

400g white cabbage, sliced

2 celery sticks, chopped

1 large red pepper, sliced

1 tbsp chopped parsley

2 garlic cloves, crushed (optional)

1 whole chilli (optional)

1 tbsp chopped dill

100ml soured cream or crème fraîche (optional)

crusty bread, to serve

Directions

STEP 1

Put the ribs in a large saucepan and pour over 3 litres cold water, then season with salt. Bring to the boil over a medium heat, skimming off any foam that rises to the surface. Peel one of the onions and add this to the pan whole, along with the beetroot. Reduce the heat to low and simmer for 1 hr-1 hr 15 mins until the meat is tender. If the ribs don't have much fat, they will need to cook for longer. Remove the whole onion and compost it.

STEP 2

Meanwhile, make zasmażka – a Ukrainian sofrito. Skim 2 tbsp fat off the ribs as they cook, and pour it into a large frying pan (or use 2 tbsp vegetable oil). Finely chop the second onion and fry it over a low-medium heat, stirring often for about 5 mins until transparent and soft. Add the grated carrots and cook for 10 mins more. Tip in the potatoes and stir in the tomato purée. Pour in the canned tomatoes and cook for 5 mins, then taste and add 1-2 tsp sugar to balance out the acidity, if needed. Add the bay leaf.

STEP 3

When the potato is soft (don't worry if it overcooks, it will give body to the borsch), add the zasmażka to the ribs and stock, and bring to the boil again. Add the cabbage, celery, pepper and parsley, and cook for 7 mins – try not to overcook the cabbage.

STEP 4

Mash the garlic, if using, with a pinch of salt to make a paste, then add this to the borsch for more flavour. Stir in the whole chilli, if using, and continue to cook briefly to warm through slightly.

STEP 5

Shred the meat using two forks and remove and discard the bones. Serve the borsch in bowls, each topped with 1 tbsp of the soured cream and some chopped dill, with some crusty bread on the side, if you like.

Chicken & pasta bake

Ingredients

2 tbsp olive oil

100g smoked streaky bacon, cut into small pieces

4 chicken breasts, cut into chunks

1 red onion, finely chopped

2 garlic cloves, finely chopped

1 red pepper, diced

1 yellow pepper, diced

1 tsp oregano

¼ tsp chilli flakes (optional)

2 x 400g cans chopped tomatoes

1 tsp caster sugar

small bunch of parsley, roughly chopped

3 tbsp mascarpone

350g pasta, any shape – if long, snap them in half

65g cheddar, grated

50g mozzarella, grated

Directions

STEP 1

Heat the oil in a large, wide casserole, over a medium heat. Stir in the bacon and cook for 5-7 mins, until crispy and browned. Remove to a bowl using a slotted spoon and set aside. Tip in the chicken and stir well to coat in the bacon fat. Turn the heat up to medium-high and cook for 3-5 mins until browned all over (it doesn't need to be cooked through at this point). Remove to the same bowl as the bacon using a slotted spoon.

STEP 2

Mix the onion and garlic in with a pinch of salt and turn the heat down to medium. Cook for 10-12 mins until softened. Add the peppers, oregano and chilli flakes, if using. Cook for a further 8-10 mins until the peppers have softened. Pour in the canned tomatoes, then swill out the cans with a little water and tip this in as well. Sprinkle over the sugar and stir in the chicken and bacon and most of the parsley. Season well and bring to a simmer. Cook for 20-25 mins, until thickened. Mix in the mascarpone, stirring well until dissolved.

STEP 3

Meanwhile, cook the pasta for 2 mins less than the pack states, then drain thoroughly reserving a mug of the pasta cooking water. Heat the oven to 220C/200C fan/gas 7. Taste and season the sauce before tipping in the cooked pasta. Pour in a splash of the pasta cooking water to bring the sauce together before spooning the mixture into an ovenproof baking dish. Will keep covered and frozen for up to three months. Defrost thoroughly in the fridge overnight before baking. Top with both cheeses and bake for 10-15 mins until golden and bubbling. Scatter over the remaining parsley and serve straight from the dish.

Classic California roll

Ingredients

50g fresh, sushi-grade salmon fillet, 1cm thick, skinned and boned (ask your fishmonger to do this for you)

1 sheet of nori

1 handful cooked sushi rice, roughly 80g

1 tbsp tobiko (flying fish roe) or masago (capelin roe), alternatively black or white sesame seeds

wasabi (optional)

½ avocado, stoned and skin removed, sliced into 1cm pieces

40g white crabmeat

Directions

STEP 1

Slice the salmon lengthways into 1cm-wide strips. Put a sheet of cling film underneath a sushi mat then put a sheet of nori onto the sushi mat, with the lines of the sheet lying horizontally across the mat. It does not matter if the shiny side is facing up or down – the nori won't be seen in the finished roll.

STEP 2

Wet your fingers slightly (damp fingers help when handling sticky sushi rice). Leave a space about 3-4cm from the bottom of the nori sheet. Spread the rice over the rest of the nori evenly and gently with your fingertips. You want roughly a 2mm layer. Do not press it onto the sheet.

STEP 3

Sprinkle 1 tbsp of tobiko, masago or sesame seeds over the rice; this will end up on the outside of the roll. Carefully flip the nori over on the mat so the rice is now underneath and the nori is face-up. Put the wasabi, if using, and salmon in a single line at the bottom of the nori on the area without the rice, then add half the avocado strips alongside, followed by the crabmeat in a line next to the avocado. It should all fit on to the clear area of nori just below the rice.

STEP 4

Holding the filling in place with your index fingers, start rolling the mat from the bottom edge of the nori towards the top of the rice edge. Keep rolling, holding the roll in place, 3 or 4 times, making sure that it's tightly rolling so that there are no gaps between the fillings and the nori.

STEP 5

Put the sushi roll on a clean, dry chopping board. Gently cut each roll into 8 pieces with a sharp, wet knife, smoothly and quickly. It's useful to keep fingers damp when handling and chopping. We recommend cleaning the knife after every cut to avoid the rice sticking.

Chicken nuggets

Ingredients

400g chicken breast fillets

4 tbsp plain flour

1 egg, lightly beaten

115g panko breadcrumbs or other dried breadcrumbs

2 tbsp vegetable or sunflower oil

Directions

STEP 1

Cut the chicken into bite-sized pieces and place the pieces between two layers of baking paper. Use a rolling pin to gently flatten the pieces until they are around 2-3mm thick and uniform.

STEP 2

Tip the flour onto a plate and mix it with a pinch of salt. Put the beaten egg in a bowl, and tip the breadcrumbs into another bowl. For the air fryer method, lightly oil a large baking tray.

STEP 3

Dip each chicken piece in the flour, then into the egg (shaking off the excess), and finally toss in the breadcrumbs. Transfer the coated chicken pieces to a lightly oiled baking tray for the oven method or the air fryer basket for the air fryer method. Breadcrumbing using one hand is less messy.

STEP 4

If you're using the oven, not pan-frying, preheat it to 220C/200C fan/gas 7. Bake the nuggets for 10-15 mins, turning them halfway through.

STEP 5

If you're using the air-fryer, preheat it to 200C for 4 mins. Brush the chicken pieces on both sides with oil. Cook the nuggets in batches in the air-fryer basket for 5 mins per batch until golden and crunchy. Shake the basket halfway through to ensure even cooking.

STEP 6

Serve the chicken nuggets with tomato sauce, if you like.

Sloppy joes

Ingredients

1tbsp vegetable oil

1 onion, finely chopped

2 small red peppers or yellow peppers, finely chopped

400g minced beef

2 x 400g cans chopped tomatoes

4tbsp Nando's PERi-BBQ sauce

4 cheese slices

6 burger buns

crispy onions, to serve

tbsp iceberg lettuce, to serve

Directions

STEP 1

Heat the oil in a deep frying pan, and tip in the mince, breaking it up with a wooden spoon as you go, until browned all over. Stir in the onion and pepper and cook for 8-10 mins until softened. Tip in the tomatoes and Nando's PERi-BBQ sauce, and season. Simmer for 20-25 mins until the sauce has thickened.

STEP 2

Put the cheese slices on top of the mince and cover with a lid for 2 mins to let it melt into the sauce. Pile into the buns with the crispy onions, and lettuce on the side for scooping up the extra sauce.

Tofu curry

Ingredients

1tbsp rapeseed oil

tofu, cut into 2cm cubes

2 red onions, thinly sliced

1½ tsp ginger and garlic paste

1½ tsp ground turmeric

400ml light coconut milk

2 limes, 1 juiced, 1 cut into wedges to serve

160g baby spinach

10g coriander, most roughly chopped, reserve a few whole leaves to serve

4 wholemeal chapatis, to serve

Directions

STEP 1

Heat 1/2 tbsp of the oil in a large, wide, non-stick frying pan over a medium-high heat. Fry the tofu with a pinch of salt for 5 mins, turning every couple of minutes until golden brown. Remove to a plate using a slotted spoon.

STEP 2

Add the remaining oil to the pan, then fry half the onions for 5 mins, stirring often until golden brown. Add the ginger and garlic paste, stir-frying for a minute, then add the turmeric and cook for another 30 seconds to release the flavour.

STEP 3

Stir in the coconut milk, then return the tofu to the pan along with the lime juice and 100ml water, and simmer for 5 mins. Stir in the spinach and the coriander, and cook for 1 min until wilted, then season.

STEP 4

Serve the curry in bowls topped with the coriander leaves and the remaining onion, the lime wedges for squeezing over, and the chapatis on the side.

Cholent

Ingredients

2 tbsp sunflower oil

1 large onion, peeled and cut into 2.5cm chunks

6 garlic cloves, finely chopped

1.2kg beef brisket, cut into 2.5cm cubes (remove sinew and excess fat)

4 medium potatoes (approx 450g), peeled and cut into 5cm chunks

1 large sweet potato (approx 250g), peeled and cut into 5cm chunks

2 parsnips (approx 225g), peeled and cut into 2cm chunks

225g carrots, peeled into 2cm chunks

400g can butter beans, drained and rinsed

400g can chickpeas, drained and rinsed

150g pearl barley

2 tbsp date syrup, or regular honey

1 tsp sweet paprika

1 tsp smoked paprika

2 tbsp tomato purée

1 tsp onion granules

Directions

STEP 1

Heat 1 tbsp of the sunflower oil in a large frying pan set over a medium-high heat and sauté the onions, stirring frequently, for 8-10 mins, until soft and translucent. Add the garlic and cook for a few minutes, until soft and fragrant. Sprinkle over 1 tbsp sugar and continue to cook for 2-3 mins, stirring frequently, until the garlic and onions are golden. Tip onto a plate and set aside.

STEP 2

Wipe the pan with kitchen paper and add the remaining oil. Season the cubed brisket with plenty of salt and pepper, and brown in batches, for 5-10 mins, until browned on all sides. Transfer the browned beef to a second plate or bowl.

Chicken chop suey

Ingredients

2 tbsp vegetable oil

1 large chicken breast, cut into thin bite-sized slices

1 onion, sliced

2 garlic cloves, roughly chopped or minced

1 carrot, sliced

½ tbsp dark soy sauce

½ tsp chicken powder or a pinch of salt

½ tsp sugar

pinch of white pepper (essential as it totally changes the flavour of the dish)

2 spring onions, chopped into slivers

100g ready-to-eat beansprouts

1 tbsp cornflour, mixed with 2 tbsp water

1 tsp sesame oil

steamed white rice or fried noodles, to serve

Directions

STEP 1

Heat a wok over a high heat and, once hot, pour in the oil. Add the chicken and fan out in a single layer so that it's in direct contact with the hot wok. Once it has started to brown on one side, give it a good stir, then toss in the onion and garlic. Stir, then add the carrots, dark soy, chicken powder or salt, sugar, white pepper and spring onions. Stir, then add the beansprouts and fry, stirring, for 1 min before pouring in 50ml just-boiled water.

STEP 2

Bring to the boil, then slowly pour in the cornflour paste to loosen it, mixing at the same time to prevent any lumps. Once the sauce has thickened, switch off the heat and add the sesame oil. Serve on a bed of steamed white rice or freshly fried noodles.

Fresh salmon with Thai noodle salad

Ingredients

2 skinless salmon fillets

1 large orange, the juice and zest of half, the rest peeled and chopped

125g French beans, trimmed and halved

50g mange tout, shredded

75g frozen peas

75g vermicelli rice noodles

2 tsp red curry paste

1 tsp fish sauce

3 spring onions, finely chopped

half a pack basil or coriander, chopped

Directions

STEP 1

Put a pan of water on to boil. Line a steamer with baking parchment, add the salmon fillets and scatter with a little of the orange zest. When the water is boiling, add the beans to the pan, put the salmon in the steamer on top and cook for 5 mins. Take the salmon off, and if it is cooked, set aside but add the peas and mange tout to the pan and cook for 1 min more, or if not quite cooked leave on top for the extra min. Drain the veg, but return the boiling water to the pan, add the noodles and leave to soak for 5 mins.

Lasagne soup

Ingredients

75g pancetta

2 tbsp olive oil

1 onion, roughly chopped

1 carrot, roughly chopped

1 celery stick, roughly chopped

3 garlic cloves, roughly chopped

250g 15% fat beef mince

1 tbsp tomato purée

1 tsp dried mixed herbs

400g can cherry tomatoes

1 litre beef stock

1 bay leaf

150g lasagne sheets, broken into shards

30g parmesan, grated

75g mascarpone

10g basil leaves, torn, to serve (optional)

Directions

STEP 1

Tip the pancetta into a large flameproof casserole dish over a low heat and cook, stirring often until all the fat has released and the pancetta is crisp and golden, about 8-10 mins. Remove to a bowl using a slotted spoon. Pour the olive oil into the dish and turn the heat up to medium. Once the oil is shimmering, cook the onion, carrot and celery for 15 mins until beginning to soften, then stir in the garlic and cook for another 2 mins.

STEP 2

Turn up the heat to medium-high, tip in the mince and cook for 3-4 mins until browned. Return the pancetta to the pan, then add the tomato purée and herbs, and cook for 2 mins more until darkened slightly.

STEP 3

Pour in the cherry tomatoes and beef stock, and stir to combine. Bring to the boil, season well, then add the bay leaf and reduce the heat to a simmer. Cook for 15-20 mins, then add the lasagne sheets and simmer for another 5 mins, stirring to break up the sheets.

STEP 4

Meanwhile, mix most of the parmesan with all of the mascarpone and plenty of seasoning, and heat the grill to high. Once the pasta is al dente and the soup is bubbling and has thickened, dot the mascarpone mixture over the soup and sprinkle over the remaining parmesan. Slide under the hot grill for 3-5 mins until the topping is golden and bubbling. Divide between four bowls and serve scattered with basil, if you like.

Beef rissoles

Ingredients

1 onion, grated

50g panko breadcrumbs

400g beef mince

1 courgette, trimmed and grated

1 carrot, grated

1 egg, beaten

1 garlic clove, crushed or finely grated

2 tsp dried mixed herbs

1 tsp Worcestershire sauce

2 tsp vegetable oil

peas and mash, to serve (optional)

Directions

STEP 1

Mix all the Ingredients, except the oil, together into a large bowl with 2 tsp each salt and pepper. Use your hands to make sure everything is well combined. Shape the mince mixture into 14-16 balls, then flatten into small burger-like patties and chill for 15 mins, if you have time (this helps the patties hold their shape).

STEP 2

Heat the oil in a frying pan over a medium-low heat and, once hot, fry the rissoles for 3-4 mins, then flip and fry for 3-4 mins more until cooked through. (You may need to do this in batches.) When ready, they should ready 65C on a meat thermometer. Serve with peas and mash, if you like.

DELECTABLE SNACK IDEAS

Rainbow rice

Ingredients

100g basmati rice, long grain rice or brown rice

1small red pepper, deseeded and finely chopped

½ cucumber, deseeded and finely chopped

1large carrot, grated

6 dried apricots, chopped

2 tbsp toasted pumpkin seed or sunflower seeds

2 tbsp olive oil

½ orange, juice only

Directions

STEP 1

Cook the rice as per pack instructions. Drain, rinse and drain again. Mix with the red pepper, cucumber, grated carrot, dried apricots and toasted pumpkin seeds. Drizzle over olive oil and the orange juice.

Quick chicken chasseur

Ingredients

8 rashers streaky bacon, chopped into large pieces

4 chicken breasts, cut into large chunks

200g pack baby button mushroom

1 tbsp plain flour

400g tin chopped tomato with garlic

1 beef stock cube

dash Worcestershire sauce

handful of parsley, chopped

Directions

STEP 1

Heat a shallow saucepan and sizzle the bacon for about 2 mins until starting to brown. Throw in the chicken, then fry for 3-4 mins until it has changed colour. Turn up the heat and throw in the mushrooms. Cook for a few mins, stir in the flour, then cook until a paste forms.

STEP 2

Tip in the tomatoes, stir, then crumble in the stock cube. Bubble everything for 10 mins, splash in the Worcestershire sauce, stir through the parsley, then serve with mash or boiled rice.

Cheddar scones

Ingredients

200g self-raising flour, plus a little more for dusting

50g butter, at room temperature

25g porridge oats

75g grated cheddar, plus extra for topping (optional)

150ml milk

To serve

avocado, soft cheese, ham, cucumber, cress

Directions

STEP 1

Heat oven to 220c/fan 200c/gas 7. Place the flour in a large bowl, then rub in the butter. Stir in the oats and cheese, then the milk – if it feels like it might be dry, add a touch more milk, then bring together to make a soft dough.

STEP 2

Lightly dust the surface with a little flour. roll out the dough no thinner than 2cm. Using a 4cm plain cutter, firmly stamp out the rounds – try not to twist the cutter as this makes the scones rise unevenly. re-roll the trimmings and stamp out more.

STEP 3

Transfer to a non-stick baking sheet, dust with a little more flour or grated cheese, then bake for 12-15 mins until well risen and golden. Cool on a wire rack before serving on their own or topped with mashed avocado, or soft cheese, and ham, cucumber or cress.

Marshmallows

Ingredients

3 large egg whites

13 leaves of gelatine

700g white caster sugar

1 ½ tbsp liquid glucose

1 vanilla pod, seeds scraped

sunflower oil for the tin

For dusting

100g icing sugar

4 tbsp cornflour

Directions

STEP 1

Whisk the egg whites in a large heat proof bowl using electric beaters. Whisk until soft peaks form then set aside. Put the gelatine in a deep bowl or jug and cover with 200ml cold water to soften.

STEP 2

Put the caster sugar, liquid glucose and 300ml water in a large, high-sided saucepan. Cook over a medium-high heat until the mixture reaches 130C on a sugar thermometer. Be very careful when you work with hot sugar. Take the pan off the heat then add the gelatine and the water they were soaked in to the hot sugar. Take care or wear oven gloves as the sugar can bubble up and spit. Stir until the gelatine has dissolved then carefully pour the mixture into a heatproof jug.

STEP 3

Return the beaters to egg whites and whip up further until stiff peaks form. Keep whisking while you slowly pour in the warm syrup in a steady stream. Keep beating the mixture until it is smooth and shiny, then add the vanilla seeds. Continue to use the electric beaters for around 8-10mins or until the mixture is noticeably thicker.

STEP 4

Line a 25cm x 35cm roasting tin (or any large and deep rectangular dish) with cling film and brush with sunflower oil. Mix the icing sugar and cornflour together then sieve a third of the mixture into the tray to coat the inside. Pour in the marshmallow mixture, level with a spatula and leave to set for 2 hours.

STEP 5

Spread a large sheet of baking parchment over your surface and sieve another third of the cornflour sugar mix over it. Upturn the set marshmallow onto the dusted sheet and peel away the cling film. Dust with a little more of the cornflour sugar and dust a large sharp knife with it too.

STEP 6

Cut the marshmallows into small squares approx. 3cm x 3cm sieving a little more cornflour sugar over all cut sides and knife as you go. You may not need all of it but they need to be coated on all sides otherwise they will stick. Serve straightway or keep in an airtight container for up to 2 days, separated with layers of baking parchment.

Crispy roasted chickpeas

Ingredients

1 x 400g can chickpeas, drained

1tsp rapeseed oil

2tsp smoked paprika

2tsp ground cumin

2tsp ground coriander

½tsp cayenne pepper

Directions

STEP 1

Heat oven to 200C/180C fan/gas 4. Tip the chickpeas into a bowl and toss with the rapeseed oil, smoked paprika, cumin and coriander along with a big pinch of salt. Toss well until the chickpeas are well coated, then tip out onto a baking tray and bake for 35 mins, moving them round the tray halfway through so they dry out evenly and are crunchy. Leave to cool, then store in an airtight container.

Rhubarb & date chutney

Ingredients

50g fresh root ginger, grated

300ml red wine vinegar

500g eating apple, peeled and finely chopped

200g pitted date, chopped

200g dried cranberries or raisins

1 tbsp mustard seed

1 tbsp curry powder

400g light muscovado sugar

700g rhubarb, sliced into 2cm chunks

500g red onion

Directions

STEP 1

Put the onions in a large pan with the ginger and vinegar. Bring to the boil, then simmer for 10 mins. Add the rest of the Ingredients, except the rhubarb, plus 2 tsp salt to the pan and bring to the boil, stirring. Simmer, uncovered, for about 10 mins until the apples are tender.

STEP 2

Stir in the rhubarb and cook, uncovered, until the chutney is thick and jammy, about 15-20 mins. Leave the chutney to sit for about 10-15 mins, then spoon into warm, clean jars, and seal. Label the jars when cool. Keep for at least a month before eating.

Air fryer tofu (popcorn nuggets)

Ingredients

1 block extra-firm tofu

4 tbsp plain flour

1½ tsp paprika

1 tsp Dijon mustard

125ml milk

75g panko breadcrumbs

½ tsp garlic granules

1 tbsp bouillon powder

Directions

STEP 1

Wrap the tofu in a clean tea towel, then put it on a large plate with a lip. Put a heavy item such as a frying pan on top and then add cans or jars to add weight. Leave for 30 mins. The tofu should shrink in size and release its liquid. Can be pressed for 24 hrs in advance.

STEP 2

Cut the tofu into 3cm squares or rip into chunks. Put into a bowl and toss with 1 tbsp flour and 1 tsp paprika. Set aside. Combine the remaining flour, Dijon mustard and milk in a bowl. Whisk if it gets a little lumpy and set aside. Mix together the breadcrumbs, garlic granules, bouillon and ½ tsp paprika in another bowl, then tip onto a tray.

Chiu Chow smacked cucumber

Ingredients

1 cucumber

1 garlic clove, finely chopped

2 tsp caster sugar

1 tbsp light soy sauce

2 tsp rice vinegar

1-2 tsp chilli oil, plus extra to serve (optional)

Directions

STEP 1

Put the cucumber on a chopping board and lightly bash it along the length using a rolling pin, or by using your fist to push down on the flat blade of a cleaver – you want to break the flesh a little but not turn it to a pulp. Cut the cucumber in half and scoop out the seeds, then cut the flesh into bite-sized pieces. Sprinkle over about ½ tsp sea salt (you can do this on the chopping board), leave for 10 mins, then rinse well in cold water and drain.

STEP 2

Mix the garlic, sugar, light soy sauce and rice vinegar with the chilli oil in a serving bowl. Add the cucumber and leave to marinade for 10 mins. Serve with more of the chilli oil on the side, if you like, for those who prefer more spice.

Loaded fries

Ingredients

1 red onion, halved and finely sliced

½ lime, juiced

450g frozen oven fries

2 tsp Cajun seasoning, plus a pinch

6 pork or chorizo-style sausages

150g mixed grated cheddar and mozzarella cheese

2 tomatoes, finely chopped

150g soured cream

50g pickled jalapeños

small bunch of coriander, leaves picked

Directions

STEP 1

Combine the sliced onion, lime juice and a pinch of salt in a non-metallic bowl, and set aside to lightly pickle for 20 mins. Will keep chilled for up to five days.

STEP 2

Heat the oven to 200C/180C fan/gas 6. Arrange the fries in a single layer over a large baking tray, sprinkle with a generous pinch of the Cajun seasoning and bake for 10 mins, shaking the tray after 5 mins. They should be cooked but not have much colour.

STEP 3

Meanwhile, squeeze the sausagemeat from the skins into a frying pan, and add the 2 tsp Cajun seasoning. Fry over a medium heat, breaking the meat up with a wooden spoon, until cooked and browned in places.

STEP 4

Remove the fries from the oven, then scatter over the cooked sausage and cheese. Return to the oven for 10 mins until the cheese has melted and the chips are golden and crisp.

STEP 5

Top the hot fries with the tomatoes, soured cream, jalapeños, pickled onions and coriander leaves just before serving.

Chocolate & raspberry pots

Ingredients

200g plain chocolate (not too bitter, 50% or less)

100g frozen raspberry, defrosted or fresh raspberries

500g Greek yogurt

3 tbsp honey

chocolate curls or sprinkles, for serving

Directions

STEP 1

Break the chocolate into small pieces and place in a heatproof bowl. Bring a little water to the boil in a small saucepan, then place the bowl of chocolate on top, making sure the bottom of the bowl does not touch the water. Leave the chocolate to melt slowly over a low heat.

STEP 2

Remove the chocolate from the heat and leave to cool for 10 mins. Meanwhile, divide the raspberries between 6 small ramekins or glasses.

STEP 3

When the chocolate has cooled slightly, quickly mix in the yogurt and honey. Spoon the chocolate mixture over the raspberries. Place in the fridge to cool, then finish the pots with a few chocolate shavings before serving.

Scrambled omelette toast topper

Ingredients

2 eggs

1 tbsp crème fraîche

25g cheddar, grated

small bunch chive, snipped

1 spring onion, sliced

1 tsp oil

3-4 cherry tomatoes, halved

2 slices crusty bread, toasted

Directions

STEP 1

Beat together eggs, crème fraîche, cheese and chives with a little seasoning. Heat oil in a pan, then soften spring onion for a few mins. Add tomatoes and warm through, then pour in egg mixture. Cook over a low heat, stirring, until eggs are just set. Pile over toast.

Classic apple chutney

Ingredients

1 ½kg cooking apples, peeled and diced

750g light muscovado sugar

500g raisins

2 medium onions, finely chopped

2 tsp mustard seeds

2 tsp ground ginger

1 tsp salt

700ml cider vinegar

Directions

STEP 1

Combine all the Ingredients in a large, heavy saucepan. Bring the mixture to a boil over a medium heat, then simmer uncovered, stirring frequently, for 30-40 mins, or until thick and pulpy. Remove from the heat, leave to cool and transfer to sterilised, clean, dry jars and seal.

Nacho chicken bake

Ingredients

300g jar mild or hot salsa, whichever you prefer

210g can red kidney beans

200g cooked chicken (leftover from a roast is ideal), chopped

0.5 small pack coriander, chopped

about 75g nacho cheese tortilla chips

75g cheddar, grated

salad, to serve

avocado, to serve

1 lime, to serve

Directions

STEP 1

Heat oven to 190C/170C fan/gas 5. Tip the jar of salsa and the beans with their juice into a pan. Stir in the chicken and coriander, then heat until bubbling.

STEP 2

Tip the mixture into a shallow ovenproof dish. Top with the tortillas and cheese, then bake for 8 mins. Serve with a salad, preferably including some avocado, and a good squeeze of lime.

Hummus without tahini

Ingredients

400g can chickpeas, drained (liquid reserved)

½ small garlic clove, crushed, or ½ tsp garlic purée

1 tsp lemon juice

2 tbsp olive oil, plus a drizzle

pittas or vegetable crudités, to serve

Directions

STEP 1

Tip the chickpeas, garlic, lemon juice and olive oil
into a small blender or food processor. Season and

add 1 tbsp of the reserved liquid from the can of chickpeas.

STEP 2

Blitz together until smooth, adding more of the reserved chickpea liquid to make a smoother hummus, if you like. Tip the hummus into a bowl, drizzle with more olive oil and chill until ready to serve. Serve with pittas or vegetable crudités.

Double chocolate shortbreads

Ingredients

175g butter, softened

85g golden caster sugar

200g plain flour

2 tbsp cocoa powder

100g chocolate chips, milk or dark

Directions

STEP 1

Mix the butter and sugar together with a wooden spoon. Stir in the flour and cocoa, followed by the chocolate chips – you'll probably need to mix it together with your hands at this stage. Halve the dough and roll each piece into a log about 5cm thick. Wrap in cling film and chill for 1 hr or for several days. Can be frozen for up to 1 month.

STEP 2

Heat oven to 180C/160C fan/gas 4. Slice logs into 1cm-thick rounds, transfer to a baking tray lined with baking parchment and bake for 10-12 mins. Cool on the tray.

DELECTABLE SOUP IDEAS

Pea & pesto soup with fish finger croûtons

Ingredients

500g frozen pea

4 medium potatoes, peeled and cut into cubes

1l hot vegetable stock

300g pack fish finger (about 10)

3 tbsp green pesto

Directions

STEP 1

Tip the peas and potatoes into a large saucepan, then pour in the stock. Bring to the boil and simmer for 10 mins, until the potato chunks are tender. Meanwhile, grill the fish fingers as per pack instructions until cooked through and golden. Cut into bitesize cubes and keep warm.

STEP 2

Take a third of the peas and potatoes out of the pan with a slotted spoon and set aside. Blend the rest of the soup until smooth, then stir in the pesto with the reserved vegetables. Heat through and serve in warm bowls with the fish finger croûtons on top.

Danish-style yellow split pea soup

Ingredients

500g dried yellow split peas, soaked for at least 2 hrs, rinsed

2 onions, finely chopped

1 large leek, finely chopped

2 medium carrots, cut into 1cm chunks

1 small celeriac, peeled and cut into 1cm chunks

2 medium parsnips, peeled and cut into 1cm chunks

2 litres fresh vegetable stock

2 tbsp sweet white miso

1 tsp caraway seeds

1 tsp white pepper, plus extra to serve

large pinch of ground cloves

6 thyme or oregano sprigs, tied

handful of fresh dill, chopped, to serve

rye bread, mustard and pickle, to serve (optional)

Directions

STEP 1

Drain the peas and bring to the boil in a pan of salted water. Cook for 10 mins, drain, rinse and put in a slow cooker with the remaining Ingredients except the dill. Cover and cook on low for 6-8 hrs, or until everything has softened. Remove and discard the thyme.

STEP 2

Stir, adjusting the soup with 250-300ml boiled water as needed. Season to taste. Sprinkle over the dill and serve with rye bread, mustard and pickle, if you like.

Cream of cauliflower soup with sautéed wild mushrooms

Ingredients

1large cauliflower (about 1.3kg/3lb), stalks discarded and florets chopped

1large potato, peeled and chopped into large chunks

1medium onion, chopped

25g butter

4 tbsp olive oil

1.2l light chicken or vegetable stock

600ml full-fat milk

142ml carton double cream

250g wild mushroom – choose from ceps, girolles (chanterelles), morels (either a mixture or just one type)

1-2 tbsp finely snipped chives

Directions

STEP 1

Put the cauliflower, potato and onion in a large saucepan with the butter and half of the oil. Gently heat the contents until they start to sizzle, then cover with a lid and sweat over a low heat for about 10 minutes, stirring occasionally. The vegetables should be softened but not coloured.

STEP 2

Pour in the stock and bring to the boil, then pour in the milk and return gently to a boil. This way, there will be no scum forming from the milk. Season to taste then simmer, uncovered, for 10-15 minutes until the vegetables are soft. Pour in half the cream.

STEP 3

Blend everything in a food processor or blender, in batches. For an extra creamy texture, push the purée through a sieve with the back of a ladle. Stir in the rest of the cream. (If preparing ahead cool, cover and chill for up to a day.)

STEP 4

To serve, pick over the mushrooms. Wild mushrooms can be gritty so wash them quickly in a bowl of cold water then drain well and pat dry. Trim the stalks and chop or slice the mushrooms neatly. Heat the remaining oil in a frying pan and, when very hot, stir fry the mushrooms quickly until nicely browned, seasoning with salt and freshly ground black pepper as you cook them.

STEP 5

Reheat the soup until piping hot. Check for seasoning and ladle into warmed bowls. Spoon the mushrooms into the centre and sprinkle lightly with the chives. Italy's elegant, mildly citrussy whites, such as Vernaccia di San Gimignano, or a Chardonnay would suit this rich soup.

Chipotle black bean soup with lime-pickled onions

Ingredients

juice 2 limes

2 small red onions, thinly sliced

½ tbsp olive oil

2 garlic cloves, finely chopped

½ tbsp ground cumin

½ tbsp smoked paprika

½ tbsp chipotle paste, or Tabasco, to taste

400g can black bean, drained and rinsed

400ml vegetable stock

half-fat soured cream, to serve

coriander leaves, to serve

crisp tortilla chips, to serve

Directions

STEP 1

To make the lime-pickled onions, combine ½ the lime juice and ½ the onions in a small bowl, and season. Leave to pickle for 30 mins.

STEP 2

Meanwhile, heat the olive oil in a saucepan over a medium-high heat. Add the garlic and remaining onions, and season. Cook for 8 mins or until the onions are translucent. Add the spices and chipotle purée, cook for 1 min, then add the beans, stock and remaining lime juice. Simmer for 15 mins, then purée in a blender.

STEP 3

Pour the soup into a clean pan to reheat. Serve with a little of the drained pickled onions, topped with a small drizzle of soured cream and some coriander, and the tortillas on the side.

Creamy chicken soup

Ingredients

1kg pack free-range chicken thigh, skin removed

300ml dry white wine

2 large onions, cut into large wedges

4 celery sticks, quartered

3 leeks, quartered

2 sprigs thyme, plus extra leaves for sprinkling

2 bay leaves

½ tsp ground white pepper (optional)

40g plain flour

300ml pot double cream

Directions

STEP 1

Put the chicken thighs in a very large, heavy-based pan and fry for a few mins, turning frequently to lightly colour them. Providing the heat is low, there is no need to add any oil. Pour in the wine, turn up the heat and boil rapidly to evaporate the alcohol. Pile in the veg and herbs, add 1 tsp salt and the white pepper (or you can use black pepper). Pour in 2 litres boiling water. Cover the pan and simmer for 45 mins until the chicken and veg are tender. Take out the bay leaves and thyme sprigs and cool for about 30 mins.

STEP 2

Remove chicken from the soup, then strip the meat from the bones. Put all but 140g of the chicken back into the pan. Blitz the soup with a hand blender or in batches in a food processor until very smooth, then return to the pan.

STEP 3

Blend the flour and cream together with a couple of ladles of the soup, then stir the creamy mixture into the rest of the soup and heat, stirring continuously until thickened. You can blitz again if it looks a little lumpy. Chop the remaining chicken and stir into the soup. Scatter with thyme leaves, to serve.

Creamy mushroom soup

Ingredients

25g dried porcini (ceps)

50g butter

1 onion, finely chopped

1 garlic clove, sliced

thyme sprigs

400g mixed wild mushrooms

850ml vegetable stock

200ml tub crème fraîche

4 slices white bread, about 100g, cubed

chives and truffle oil, to serve

Directions

STEP 1

Bring a kettle to the boil, then pour the water over
the dried porcini just to cover. Heat half the butter
in a saucepan, then gently sizzle the onion, garlic
and thyme for 5 mins until softened and starting
to brown. Drain the porcini, reserving the juice,

then add to the onion with the mixed wild mushrooms. Leave to cook for 5 mins until they go limp.

STEP 2

Pour over the stock and the reserved juices, bring to the boil, then simmer for 20 mins. Stir in crème fraîche, then simmer for a few mins more. Blitz the soup with a hand blender or liquidiser, pass through a fine sieve, then set aside.

Spiced red lentil soup

Ingredients

1 onion, chopped

1 tbsp olive oil

1-2 tbsp Thai red curry paste

300g red lentil

1.7l vegetable stock

200ml coconut milk

chopped spring onions, to serve (optional)

Directions

STEP 1

Fry the onion in 1 tbsp olive oil until soft. Stir in the red Thai curry paste, depending how hot you want it.

STEP 2

Add red lentils and mix to coat in the paste. Pour over vegetable stock and simmer for 20 mins until the lentils are tender.

STEP 3

Blend with coconut milk and reheat if needed. Serve scattered with chopped spring onions, if you like.

Minestrone in minutes

Ingredients

1l hot vegetable stock

400g tin chopped tomato

100g thin spaghetti, broken into short lengths

350g frozen mixed vegetable

4 tbsp pesto

drizzle of olive oil

coarsely grated vegetarian parmesan-style cheese,
to serve

Directions

STEP 1

Bring the stock to the boil with the tomatoes, then add the spaghetti and cook for 6 mins or until done. A few minutes before the pasta is ready, add the vegetables and bring back to the boil. Simmer for 2 mins until everything is cooked.

STEP 2

Serve in bowls drizzled with pesto and oil, sprinkled with parmesan.

Prawn & fennel bisque

Ingredients

450g raw tiger prawn in their shells

4 tbsp olive oil

1 large onion, chopped

1 large fennel bulb, chopped, fronds reserved

2 carrots, chopped

150ml dry white wine

1 tbsp brandy

400g can chopped tomato

1l fish stock

2 generous pinches paprika

To serve

150ml pot double cream

8 tiger prawns, shelled, but tail tips left on (optional)

fennel fronds (optional)

Directions

STEP 1

Shell the prawns, then fry the shells in the oil in a large pan for about 5 mins. Add the onion, fennel and carrots and cook for about 10 mins until the veg start to soften. Pour in the wine and brandy, bubble hard for about 1 min to drive off the alcohol, then add the tomatoes, stock and paprika.

Cover and simmer for 30 mins. Meanwhile, chop the prawns.

STEP 2

Blitz the soup as finely as you can with a stick blender or food processor, then press through a sieve into a bowl. Spend a bit of time really working the mixture through the sieve as this will give the soup its velvety texture.

Moroccan spiced cauliflower & almond soup

Ingredients

1 large cauliflower

2 tbsp olive oil

½ tsp each ground cinnamon, cumin and coriander

2 tbsp harissa paste, plus extra drizzle

1l hot vegetable or chicken stock

50g toasted flaked almond, plus extra to serve

Directions

STEP 1

Cut the cauliflower into small florets. Fry olive oil, ground cinnamon, cumin and coriander and harissa paste for 2 mins in a large pan. Add the cauliflower, stock and almonds. Cover and cook for 20 mins until the cauliflower is tender. Blend soup until smooth, then serve with an extra drizzle of harissa and a sprinkle of toasted almonds.

Easy green vegetable soup

Ingredients

1bunch spring onions, chopped

1large potato, peeled and chopped

1 garlic clove, crushed

1l vegetable stock

250g frozen peas

100g fresh spinach

300ml natural yogurt

few mint leaves, basil leaves, cress or a mixture, to
serve

Directions

STEP 1

Put the spring onions, potato and garlic into a large pan. Pour over the vegetable stock and bring to the boil.

STEP 2

Reduce the heat and simmer for 15 mins with a lid on or until the potato is soft enough to mash with the back of a spoon.

STEP 3

Add the peas and bring back up to a simmer. Scoop out around 4 tbsp of the peas and set aside for the garnish.

STEP 4

Stir the spinach and yogurt into the pan, then carefully pour the whole mixture into a blender or use a stick blender to blitz it until it's very smooth. Season to taste with black pepper.

STEP 5

Ladle into bowls, then add some of the reserved cooked peas and scatter over your favourite soft herbs or cress. Serve with crusty bread, if you like.

Chickpea tagine soup

Ingredients

2 red peppers

1 tbsp rapeseed oil

1 red onion, thinly sliced

2 large garlic cloves, crushed

2 tsp ground coriander

1 tsp ground cumin

2 tbsp rose harissa paste

2 x 400g cans chickpeas, drained and rinsed

1 ½l low-salt veg stock

150g kale, chopped

1 lemon, zested and juiced

50g dried apricots, finely chopped

1/2 small bunch parsley, finely chopped

fat-free natural yogurt, to serve (optional)

Directions

STEP 1

Heat the grill to its highest setting. Halve and deseed the peppers, then lay cut-side down on a baking sheet lined with foil. Grill for 10-15 mins, or until blistered and softened. Leave until cool enough to handle, then remove and discard the skins. Slice the roasted peppers into thin strips.

STEP 2

Heat the oil in a large saucepan over a low heat. Fry the onion for 8-10 mins until softened. Stir through the garlic, coriander, cumin and harissa paste and cook for 1 min more. Add the chickpeas and stock, bring to the boil and simmer for 15 mins, covered.

Spiced parsnip & cauliflower soup

Ingredients

1 tbsp olive oil

1 medium cauliflower, cut into florets

3 parsnips, chopped

2 onions, chopped

1 tbsp fennel seed

1 tsp coriander seed

½ tsp turmeric

3 garlic cloves, sliced

1-2 green chillies, deseeded and chopped

5cm piece ginger, sliced

zest and juice 1 lemon

1l vegetable stock

handful coriander, chopped

Directions

STEP 1

Heat the oil in a large saucepan and add the vegetables. Cover partially and sweat slowly for 10-15 mins until soft but not brown. In a separate pan, dry-roast the spices with a pinch of salt for a few mins until fragrant. Grind with a pestle and mortar to a fine powder.

STEP 2

Add the garlic, chilli, ginger and spices to the vegetables, and cook for about 5 mins, stirring regularly. Add the lemon zest and juice. Pour in the stock, topping up if necessary to just cover the veg. Simmer for 25-30 mins until all the vegetables are tender.

Honeyed carrot soup

Ingredients

2 tbsp butter

2 small leeks, sliced

800g carrots, roughly chopped

2 tsp clear honey

small pinch dried chilli flakes (optional)

1 bay leaf

2 ½l vegetable stock

soured cream or yogurt, to serve

Directions

STEP 1

Melt the butter in a large saucepan over a medium heat. Add the leeks to the pan, then cook for 3 mins until starting to soften. Add the carrots, honey, chilli (if using) and bay leaf, then cook for 2 mins.

STEP 2

Pour in the stock, bring to the boil, then simmer for 30 mins. Blend the soup in batches, return to a clean pan, then season to taste. When ready to serve, bring back to a simmer, then ladle into mugs. Add a swirl of soured cream or yogurt and serve with garlic bread or bacon butties.

Healthy mushroom soup

Ingredients

30g dried porcini mushrooms

1½ tbsp olive oil

20g unsalted butter

250g mushrooms, roughly chopped

1 medium carrot, peeled and finely diced

1 celery stick, finely diced

200g pearl barley

800ml chicken, beef or veal stock

small bunch of dill, leaves chopped

soured cream and crusty bread, to serve

Directions

STEP 1

Cover the porcini mushrooms with 750ml boiling water and leave to soak.

STEP 2

Heat the olive oil and butter in a large saucepan and add the chopped mushrooms, carrot and celery. Fry over a medium-high heat for around 10 mins or until the carrots are beginning to turn dark gold. Add the barley and stir the mixture for about

2 mins, then pour in the stock.

STEP 3

Drain the porcini, retaining the soaking liquor, and cut up any large bits. Add these to the pan, along with the liquor. Bring to the boil, then turn the heat down and simmer for 30 mins (it might take a bit longer) until the barley is tender. Taste for seasoning. Stir in the dill. Serve with a dollop of soured cream on top of each bowlful and crusty bread on the side.

CHAPTER FIVE: TO SUM UP!

A balanced diet combined with enzyme replacement therapy can help ease your symptoms and improve your quality of life. To achieve a balanced diet in your meal planning, you should:

Eat a varied diet

Since your body has difficulty absorbing nutrients, it's extra important that you choose foods with a balanced mix of:

proteins

carbohydrates

fats

A diet rich in vegetables and fruits is a great place to start.

Seek out minimally processed foods

Cooking from scratch will help you avoid processed foods and deep fried foods, which often contain hydrogenated oils that'll be hard for you to digest.

Stay hydrated

Drinking enough water will help your digestive system run smoothly. If you have diarrhea caused by EPI, it'll also prevent dehydration.

Plan ahead

Planning ahead for meals and snacks on the go will make it easier to avoid foods that aggravate your digestive system.

Lifestyle adjustments for better digestion and overall health

The right diet is very important for managing EPI. A dietitian can help you choose the foods that keep your energy level up and give you the nutrition you need. Here are a few tips:

Eat six small meals per day: Try that instead of the traditional three. A big meal might not be appealing if you have digestion troubles from EPI.

Don't drink or smoke: Alcohol can make it even harder for your body to absorb fat, and can damage your pancreas over time. Alcoholism is one possible cause of EPI. Smoking can lead to calcium buildup in your pancreas.

Take vitamins: You may need to take vitamins A, D, E, and K to replace ones that aren't getting absorbed from your diet. EPI makes it hard for you to get the right nutrients because your body can't break down your foods. You also probably don't take in enough fats. Your doctor can prescribe vitamin supplements to help you get the right levels of these nutrients. They can also tell you which over-the-counter supplements and what dosage to take.

Strategies for managing symptoms

You can manage the symptoms of EPI by taking enzyme replacements and following an eating plan that gives you the right nutrition. Make sure you get the advice of a dietitian or nutritionist. One of your big challenges is to make sure you don't lose weight. A nutritionist can help you choose foods that have enough protein and nutrients.

Also, talk with your family and friends to get the support you need while you're getting treatment. Ask your doctor about support groups, which let you talk to others who are going through the same things you are.